RADIOACTIVE BABY
Josep

Published by Joseph J. Mangano
Radiation and Public Health Project, New York NY

Printed by Lightning Source Inc., LaVergne TN

2008

Library of Congress Cataloging-in-Publishing Data

Mangano, Joseph J., 1956-

This book contains information obtained from authentic and highly regarded sources. Reprinted material is quoted with permission, and sources are indicated. A wide variety of references are listed. Reasonable efforts have been made to publish reliable data and information, but the author/publisher cannot assume responsibility for the validity of all materials or for the consequences of their use.

Neither this book nor any part may be reproduced or transmitted in any form or by any means, electronic or mechanical, including photocopying, microfilming, and recording, or by any information storage or retrieval system, without prior permission in writing from the author/publisher.

Direct all inquiries to Joseph J. Mangano, 716 Simpson Avenue, Ocean City NJ 08226.

© Copyright 2008 by Joseph J. Mangano
ISBN 13 Number 978-0-615-16875-3

CONTENTS

Acknowledgements   3

Preface   5

I. INTRODUCTION

    1. Buried Treasure – Old St. Louis Baby Teeth Discovered   7

    2. Cancer Victims Seek Cause, Not Just Cure   19

II. NUCLEAR WEAPONS TEST FALLOUT

    3. Cold War Brings Citizens and Scientists Together   27

    4. St. Louis Tooth Study of Bomb Test Fallout – Early Years   40

    5. St. Louis Study Shapes Policy in Depths of Cold War   52

    6. St. Louis Tooth Study - Later Year   63

III. NUCLEAR REACTOR EMISSIONS

    7. Reactors Rekindle Interest in Radiation Health   73

    8. U.S. Reactors Cause Child Health Concerns   83

    9. The Tooth Fairy Project Challenges U.S. Reactors   94

    10. The Tooth Fairy Project in New Jersey   109

    11. The Tooth Fairy Project Evokes Strong Reactions   122

IV. IMPACT OF BABY TOOTH STUDIES

    12. Tooth Studies - Links with Child Cancer and Legacies   135

    Reference   148

ACKNOWLEDGEMENTS

Thanks are owed to many who made preparation of this book possible. Long before this writing, those scientists who understood the health threat posed by man-made radioactive chemicals from atomic bomb tests – most notably Dr. Linus Pauling and Dr. Andrei Sakharov - brought about studies of radioactive Strontium-90 in baby teeth. The idea was originally proposed by Dr. Herman Kalckar in an August 1958 article in the journal *Nature,* and later that year, the St. Louis-based Committee for Nuclear Information and Washington University began a landmark 12-year study, largely done through volunteers.

The innovation of Dr. Jay Gould and Dr. Ernest Sternglass revived the study of Strontium-90 in baby teeth, for nuclear reactor emissions. Working side by side with these visionary men in our group's "Tooth Fairy Project" has inspired me, and others, to vigorously pursue the truth behind health threats of nuclear power. The lab work of Dr. Hari Sharma, a radiochemist at the University of Waterloo, turned the Gould/Sternglass idea into reality. Jerry Brown, Bill McDonnell, and Dr. Janette Sherman, my colleagues at the Radiation and Public Health Project, helped make the study a success.

Those scientists who maintained that health risks of even the lowest doses of radiation exposure needed to be studied deserve special praise – especially those who caused the fury of the nuclear industry and government. These include (in addition to some already mentioned) Drs. Rosalie Bertell, John Gofman, Carl Johnson, Thomas Mancuso, Karl Morgan, William Reid, Alice Stewart, Arthur Tamplin, and Steven Wing).

I much appreciate the stories recounted to me by people who worked on the St. Louis tooth study years ago. They include Dr. John Fowler, Dr. Michael Friedlander, Sophie Goodman, Yvonne Logan, Dr. Louise Reiss, and the late Harold Rosenthal.

Thanks also go to the many citizens and public leaders who brought our tooth study to the table in the discussion of nuclear reactors. Prominent among these is Alec Baldwin, who probably collected at least half of the 5,000 teeth through personal appearances and mail solicitations. Margo Frances dressed up as the tooth fairy and played guitar at many Westchester County public events. Barbara Bailine also dressed up as the tooth fairy and appeared throughout central New Jersey.

Members of the Long Island group Standing for Truth About Radiation (STAR), including Christie Brinkley and Scott Cullen, successfully lobbied the Suffolk County (NY) legislature for funds to support the tooth study. Legislators who have worked to fund the study include Matt Ahearn and Reid Gusciora in New Jersey; Ginny Fields and Tom Abinanti in New York; Bruce Smith in Pennsylvania; and Jim O'Rourke in Connecticut.

Agnes Reynolds made many calls and sent many emails to people across the nation with a child with cancer. Deirdre Imus sent a written appeal to New Jersey youngsters with cancer in the Tomorrow Children's Fund. Dr. Lewis Cuthbert and his wife Donna encouraged many in southeast Pennsylvania to donate teeth.

Credit is given to parents who donated their child's baby tooth so that its Strontium-90 level could be measured, both in St. Louis in the 1960s and in the U.S. since the late 1990s. Special credit goes to parents of nearly 200 children with cancer, whose donation of a tooth signified their interest in finding out more about one potential cause of cancer. One of these children, Cory Furst of New Jersey, made several public presentations about his battle with cancer and the tooth study as one means of finding causes of the disease.

Thanks go to Dr. Barry Commoner of Queens College, who recommended that St. Louis baby teeth discovered in 2001 be given to our group for further study; to Dr. Danny Kohl of Washington University in St. Louis, who arranged for the donation of the teeth, and to RPHPs Marsha Marks, who supervised the transfer of the teeth. In addition, the 2000 St. Louis "Baby Boomers" and their parents who wrote our organization in support of a follow up health study should be commended for seeking answers to the cancer menace.

Tim Jones of the Louis and Harold Price Foundation, along with David Friedson and Gail Merrill, are to be singled out for recognizing the importance of the study of Strontium-90 in baby teeth.

And last but not least, the book could not have been possible without the help and encouragement of my dear wife Susan, who I met while working on the tooth study. She steadfastly believes in the importance of this work as a means of keeping our society's children healthy.

Joseph J. Mangano
Ocean City NJ
October 18, 2007

PREFACE

The study of Strontium-90 levels in baby teeth was the result of two forces colliding.

The first was the explosion in cancer rates, especially in children, during the 20th century. The rate of the disease in youngsters (and adults) has nearly doubled since the 1940s. But among cancer sufferers, there is a special shock value for children as innocent victims. The human mind cannot easily rationalize a 10 year old with leukemia, compared to, for example, a 78 year old man with prostate cancer. Children have not had a chance to experience much of life. They cannot be blamed for cancer, as they don't smoke, drink, or have poor personal habits. The horror of cancer in young children has translated into the building of child cancer centers and the acceleration in research to find therapies. Even though there has been relatively little attention paid to finding causes, childhood cancer gets attention.

The second was the introduction of man-made radiation into the environment. Testing atomic bombs at a furious pace in the 1950s and 1960s, with massive clouds full of radioactive chemicals was horrifying enough. But the next step (fallout entering the human body and food chain) raised even greater concerns about whether our leaders were knowingly poisoning their own people. And while all humans are harmed by radiation, the greatest harm is to fetuses, infants, and children. This concern continued after above-ground bomb testing stopped and nuclear reactors began operating, as the same toxic mix of radioactive chemicals were being released into the air and water.

Both scientists and citizens raised the obvious issues from nuclear weapons and reactors. How much radiation was entering children's bodies? Was it making them sick? There were many ways to address these questions, but studying concentrations of radioactive Strontium-90 in baby teeth became the method most commonly used. Collecting samples (donating a baby tooth that has been shed naturally) is much less invasive, cumbersome, and costly than blood or urine samples, biopsies, or autopsies. Strontium-90 has a physical half life of 29 years, meaning it decays very slowly, so that the chemical can still be detected in teeth through lab testing many years after the tooth is lost. And Strontium-90 does not exist in nature – it only is produced in atomic bomb explosions and nuclear reactor operations.

Not surprisingly, studying Strontium-90 in baby teeth became a political, as well as a scientific, issue. The race for superiority in nuclear weapons was a matter of utmost national security in which political leaders ignored or denied any health risks. Nuclear reactors were multi-billion dollar operations of utility companies unwilling to admit their product might be harming people. Resistance was not always benign, including methods that attempted to destroy the credibility of scientists and citizens searching for answers.

The attempt to combine the understanding of childhood cancer and in-body radiation has come a long way, but is far from over. There is a danger that this knowledge may never be acquired. The tools are available, but the desire to learn must overcome any resistance to this learning.

CHAPTER 1
BURIED TREASURE – OLD ST. LOUIS BABY TEETH DISCOVERED

On a warm June day in 2001, Joe Mangano sat in his office, located in his New York City apartment. The day was proceeding normally when the phone rang in the afternoon. It was Danny Kohl, a biology professor at Washington University in St. Louis. Mangano was a researcher with the group Radiation and Public Health Project (RPHP). He had been in touch with Kohl, who had been a faculty member at Washington University for over 40 years.

The call was quite unremarkable, in the minds of both Kohl and Mangano. Kohl had gotten word from university officials who contacted him as they looked for storage space. "The University has boxes of teeth" revealed Kohl, at Tyson Valley, a World War II gunnery range near St. Louis, now owned by the school. Mangano knew this meant baby teeth left over from the landmark study of radioactive Strontium-90 from atomic bomb tests in bodies. The study led to passage of the treaty that halted bomb tests above the ground, but had ended in 1970. Kohl had first phoned Barry Commoner, a biology professor who had directed the study, to ask if he was interested in the teeth. Commoner replied that he wasn't, but that Mangano's group, the Radiation and Public Health Project, should be contacted, since it was conducting another study of baby teeth of children living near nuclear reactors.

Mangano wanted to know how many teeth were at the site, and Kohl answered

> "I don't really know. I'll drive out soon to check them out, and maybe I'll take Rosenthal with me" (referring to Harold Rosenthal, who ran the laboratory that tested baby teeth in the 1960s. Rosenthal had retired but still lived in St. Louis).

The phone call ended after no more than ten minutes. Mangano resumed his work, thinking the discovery was interesting, but nothing more. That all changed the following day when Kohl phoned Mangano again, and took away Mangano's breath with what he revealed:

> "I went to Tyson Valley, and there are probably 200 cardboard boxes that look like long shoe boxes, each filled with maybe 100 teeth.

They're in this storage bunker. Some are moldy, but they haven't fallen apart. The boxes are in good shape. I took one with me to examine, they are teeth from people born in 1956."

Unlike the day before, Mangano's eyes widened. This was big, big news, a jackpot. There were thousands, maybe tens of thousands of teeth that hadn't been used in the old study, quietly slumbering away for over three decades. Washington University wasn't interested in them, and if there had been no takers, they would have thrown them away. When Kohl asked if RPHP was interested in the teeth, Mangano responded with a "my God, yes." His mind began to race. The teeth could still be tested for Strontium-90. The tooth donors weren't children any more, but in their 40s. This could mean an incredible health study, tracking the health of St. Louis kids who had donated teeth, to see if those with high Sr-90 levels as children were more likely to have died or developed cancer by middle age.

This kind of health study is known as a prospective, or longitudinal study, considered the gold standard of health research. Humans are identified for risk factors and their health is tracked over time. Probably the most famous prospective study is the Framingham heart disease study. In 1948, federal officials signed up 5,000 residents of the Massachusetts town bearing the study's name. As time went on, researchers began to see that those with heart disease were more likely to be smokers, overweight, sedentary, and have high-fat diets. These patterns held up over 50 years, for both men and women. Much of what scientists know about heart disease risk today is from the Framingham study.

The big problem with prospective studies like Framingham is that they often take many years and require large sums of money. As a result, not many are attempted. But the St. Louis teeth offered a chance for an "instant" prospective study that would be much less costly than others. Tooth donors hadn't been followed since they gave their teeth, but death records and health histories could provide the same information as if they had been continually tracked. The ability to detect levels of Strontium-90 (or other slow-decaying radioactive chemicals) would allow "high-risk" and "low-risk" children to be identified. And with thousands of teeth, significant samples would not be hard to obtain.

Things began to happen quickly. Mangano phoned his colleagues at RPHP, including Jay Gould, Ernest Sternglass, and Bill McDonnell. As the excitement spread within the group, each was sworn to silence: not a word was to be breathed. After all, they were still the property of Washington University. Moreover, nobody knew if the health study was feasible, until it was determined that either death records or health histories of tooth donors were needed.

The first step was to get the teeth. Ralph Quatrano, the chairman of the University's biology department, agreed to release the teeth to RPHP, and to pay for the shipping. RPHP supporter Marcia Marks volunteered to go to St. Louis and supervise the packing. Marks was a social worker who lived in Maryland who had taken an interest in RPHPs work. She had grown up in St. Louis and returned periodically to visit family. In a grueling effort on a hot July day, she made sure the movers placed the teeth boxes in bigger boxes, and that they were sent to McDonnell, who was to store the teeth in his office. Marks recalls that day:

> "The bunker was made of cinder blocks, and there was a musty smell to the room. But the boxes were in good shape, except the ones that touched the floor, which were somewhat mildewed."

Most boxes were sent to McDonnell, who had the space to store them, but 12 were sent separately to Mangano, just in case the unthinkable happened and the teeth were damaged or lost. They arrived safe and sound, however, and Mangano and McDonnell began to dig through the boxes. The biggest finding was that Kohl's estimate was very, very low - the actual number was 85,000 or more. McDonnell estimated that about 90% of the teeth were persons born 1954-1963, with 55% born in 1958, 1959, and 1960. Probably 95% or more had cards attached to the teeth with information identifying the donor that was legible, thus making it possible to use the teeth in a research project.

The visual effects of old 3 x 5 cards paper-clipped to small manila envelopes were strong, like going back into time. When the 86 year old Gould was hospitalized shortly after the teeth were sent from St. Louis, Mangano paid a visit and brought along some teeth. Gould was in a downcast mood, feeling trapped in his hospital bed. But when Mangano produced several teeth envelopes and cards, Gould's eyes bulged and his jaw dropped. "Oh my" he said over and over as he handled the teeth, before breaking into a hearty laugh.

Mangano and Gould attended a board meeting of Standing for Truth About Radiation, the Long Island anti-nuclear group. Mangano made a brief presentation, and passed around several tooth envelopes and cards for board members to examine. Model Christie Brinkley, a member of the group's board, immediately saw an opportunity. She began posing with the teeth, in a parody of modeling, as a camera snapped pictures and everyone laughed.

Despite all the excitement, RPHP had work to do before making the discovery public. In particular, was it possible to do a health study in which tooth donor's health history could be followed up? The first question was whether it was possible to find which donors were deceased. The results were positive. The National Center for Health Statistics informed Mangano that it kept records of all deaths in the U.S. beginning in 1979, including the name of the deceased, date of death, and cause of death. All that was needed to locate someone who died was their first and last names (maiden name for women), date of birth, and parent names – each of which was on the cards attached to tooth envelopes. If RPHP wanted to spend less money, the state of Missouri also kept records of all deaths beginning in 1979, for deaths that occurred in Missouri.

Deaths alone might make a good follow up study. About 5% of the baby boomers who were young children in the 1960s had died by their late 40s, about 7% of the males and 3% of the females. But a substantial number of these were from causes that had nothing to do with radiation exposure, like accidents, homicide, and suicide. What about those who were still alive but suffering from cancer or other diseases? There were probably as many cancer survivors as there were cancer deaths. To find out which tooth donors were sick, they needed to be contacted at their current address.

Before the Internet was invented, it probably would have been impossible to find these people. But now, companies could take a person's name and birth date and locate their current address. Gould financed a trial in which 100 St. Louis tooth donors were randomly selected and a search firm attempted to find them. The search for girls did not turn out well, probably due to the fact that many had married and changed their name since they had donated a tooth. But there was good success with boys, as a current address was produced for 82% of them.

RPHP then mailed a draft survey to these boys, asking if their birth date and parents names were correct, and if they would be willing to participate in a follow up survey. About 35% responded, all indicating the information was correct and that they would be glad to join such a survey. RPHP believed the 35% figure could be boosted; there was nothing on the return address to indicate the letter had to do with the baby teeth survey, so some may have dismissed it as junk mail and thrown it away. In addition, letters were sent while the country was in the midst of a panic after deadly anthrax was sent to Congress through the mail in the wake of the 9/11 terrorist attacks.

The final step before going public was to see if Sr-90 could be detected in the teeth. McDonnell sent a sample of teeth to radiochemist Hari Sharma, who had been testing teeth for the RPHP study in his laboratory. McDonnell deliberately did not tell Sharma that these teeth were over 40 years old, only that they were baby teeth. Using the study protocol of testing each tooth for about seven hours to get as accurate a reading as possible, Sharma came up with an accurate Sr-90 measurement for the majority of them. Some readings were inaccurate because of the lack of healthy enamel.

There was also the possibility of testing for other radioactive chemicals aside from Sr-90 in the St. Louis baby teeth. One lab advised that Plutonium-239 could be detected, and with a half life of 24,000 years, virtually all of it from the bomb tests would still be in the teeth. This gave RPHP another option for a health study.

With all preliminary questions answered, the health study was now feasible. And RPHP decided to let the country know about the discovery of the treasure of teeth.

In early November, the St. Louis Post-Dispatch was contacted. This was the same newspaper that had covered the tooth study throughout the 1960s. And even though the project had ended years ago, its editors hadn't forgotten its importance, or the sense of pride it instilled in the city. On November 9, with the nation focused almost exclusively on the terrorism issue, the Post-Dispatch nonetheless placed a long article squarely in the middle of page one. The story began with the theme of a treasure hunt:

> "Washington University researchers on a spring cleaning mission in May swung open the door to a dark, musty ammunition bunker in southwest St. Louis County and re-discovered a scientific gold mine."

The article went on to describe the opportunity to perform a follow-up health study on tooth donors. It quoted Harold Rosenthal as saying "we still don't know the effect of that on health," referring to atomic bomb test fallout.

The Post-Dispatch had its scoop, and the story hit the Associated Press wires and spread like wildfire through the U.S. media. All four major St. Louis television stations covered it, as did KMOX and other radio stations in the city. Newspapers from many cities wrote articles, including the Denver Post, Las Vegas Review Journal, Los Angeles Times, Omaha World Herald, Pittsburgh Post-Gazette, Salt Lake City Tribune, San Diego Union Tribune, San Francisco Chronicle, and Washington Post. Gould was interviewed by National Public Radio, and the British Broadcasting Company aired a story. In January, USA Today, with the largest circulation of any daily U.S. newspaper, published a lengthy article.

The San Francisco Chronicle even published an editorial supporting the idea of a follow-up health study.

> "After World War II, the United States exploded 100 nuclear bombs above ground, mostly in Nevada. At the time, peace activists – then discredited as Nervous Nellies – worried that strontium-90, a byproduct of nuclear testing, might pollute children's milk... Now workers at Washington University in St. Louis have unearthed those long-forgotten baby teeth. The New York-based Radiation and Public Health Project is attempting to find the adults who once donated them to science.
>
> There is a lesson here: Nervous Nellies who warn of environmental and health risks may drive government officials crazy, but they are not always wrong."

Most, but not all of the publicity was positive. The Washington Post article was headlined "Revival of Baby Teeth Study Denounced: Bid to Explore Effects of '60s Radiation on Donors in Later Years Called 'Junk Science'." But by and large, most of the coverage was an exciting account of the discovery and prospects for a health study.

The Post-Dispatch article included RPHPs address, phone number, and email address for those interested in the follow up study. The response was overwhelming, as 1900 emails flooded the group over the next three months, along with another 200 letters and 100 phone calls. Most were from the Baby Boomers who had donated teeth years before, or from their parents. The memories came flooding back and many recounted stories of how they gave teeth years earlier, and how they received buttons saying "I Gave My Tooth to Science."

> "A picture on the front page of the St. Louis Post-Dispatch caught my eye this morning. It was a little drawing of a kid missing some teeth with the words 'I gave my tooth to science.' I have a button just like that! I think I may be one of the donors of the 85,000 baby teeth that were collected and recently found at Washington University."

Some former residents of St. Louis who lived across the country wrote to RPHP after reading about the discovery of the teeth:

> "Wow!!! I clearly remember my mother donating every baby tooth of mine from the time that I began losing them back in 1958. (I remember it vividly because I would get so angry at my mom for sending them off)! ... It is so funny too, at my last class reunion, many of us talked about this very same thing. You can imagine my surprise when I read the article about your discovery this morning in the Fresno Bee."

A number of respondents, some of whom were researchers or scientists, immediately saw the possibility and importance of doing a follow up health study for tooth donors:

> "I understand the huge task in front of you and wish you well on your search for funding. Your project is fascinating and I think it is of tremendous importance while so many of us are still alive to discuss our health problems with you. Good luck and happy hunting!"

> "I am a physicist at Princeton University now working on technical arms control and nonproliferation issues ... We were just discussing the famous 'baby teeth' controversy in class today, so I thought it quite a coincidence to see the USA Today article."

But by far the most heartfelt correspondence came from those Baby Boomers who were suffering from cancer or other diseases, or had lost a loved one to cancer at an early age. About 130 emails and letters were of this type. A sampling of some of these responses follows. The most common type of cancer reported was thyroid cancer, which is strongly linked with radioactive iodine in bomb test fallout:

> "When I was 18 years old I came down with papillary carcinoma of the thyroid. At the time I was told it was very rare for an 18 year old to develop the disease. I wonder, after I read the article in today's paper, if my cancer came from nuclear testing."

> "I have a keen interest in this because my son, born 1958, developed thyroid cancer about 20 years later, and I've had a hunch for a long time that the radioactive fallout had something to do with it."

> "I am very interested in the tooth study, even if you don't find any of my (six) children's teeth. It is significant that two of them have had thyroid cancer."

> "Glad you are doing this… One sister and I had thyroid cancer of the type caused by exposure to external radiation. We have eliminated all possible sources, dentists, shoe measurements, genetic predisposition, etc. – except the fallout."

> "My daughter Kathleen (who died of thyroid cancer in 2000) was convinced that the large number of her friends in the 50 year old age group suffering from cancer, would have to have some common exposure to some carcinogenic agent."

> "I am very interested to hear the results of the study. I was diagnosed with breast cancer in 1996 at age 35 and then again in 2000 at age 39. I had genetic testing done to see if I have the BRCA 1 or the BRCA 2 gene , and it was inconclusive… I have no family history of breast cancer."

> "My older sister Ann Lynn died of Lymphoma in 1995. Since the family had no history of cancer, the doctors thought she may have contracted the disease through the 'environment.' Since I read your article, I wonder if it could have been caused by fallout."

> "My (first) husband was born in 1959, and was diagnosed with Mylo-monocytic Leukemia in 1989, sadly he died after a 3 year

battle. He was a strong athletic man. I guess we are all still looking for answers… if there are any. He left behind 3 children."

"I've lived in St. Louis all my life. I have come down with chronic lymphocytic leukemia and have always wondered if it came from the milk and strontium 90 which we heard a lot about back then or fallout from the A bombs. It would be interesting research to me."

"My oldest sister was diagnosed with non-Hodgkins Lymphoma in 1990 and died in 1995. We also have other instances of cancer in our family. I had heard that there are no genetic factors that would explain the lymphoma in our family, so I have to wonder if it is environmental."

"I was born in 1951 in St. Louis… I remember receiving a little button with a gap tooth smiling boy with 'I gave my tooth to science.' In 1991 I was diagnosed with squamous cell cancer of the left tonsil… I was told I had the tonsils of a 60 year old smoker and I've never smoked or drank in my life. I've had a suspicion for a long time that this had been more 'environmental' in nature."

Other letters were from people who did not have cancer, but suspected that bomb fallout may have harmed them.

"I would be interested in helping with any survey you might need. I have some autoimmune problems which are currently unexplained. Maybe someday a connection might be found."

"My sister… has had serious problems with her thyroid and had it removed approximately 5 years ago. Nobody else in the family has experienced any problems. I think that there may be a correlation between her health problems and the subject(s) that you are looking into."

"I have Hashimoto thyroiditis which is when the body thinks the thyroid is a foreign body and starts attacking it – I wonder if there is any correlation between that and the strontium 90?"

Not surprisingly, there was criticism of any potential health study – even though RPHP had not yet agreed on how to proceed. Physicist Dade

Moeller, a long time critic of the group, wasted no time in pouncing. "They have an agenda to pursue, and they will leave nothing undone to achieve their goals," he proclaimed. Stephen Musolino, a physicist who worked at Brookhaven National Laboratories, said "Their aim is well known; they dislike anything nuclear."

But these critics were overwhelmed by public support for a study of St. Louis baby tooth donors. It seemed almost certain that a follow up study would be funded. Years earlier, Gould had received support for his first book *Deadly Deceit* from the Deer Creek Foundation, a St. Louis charity that funded liberal causes. RPHP placed an application to Deer Creek, proposing to study a sample of the St. Louis tooth donors. A number of people who were leaders of the study 40 years ago sent in letters of support.

One day Mangano received a phone call from Deer Creek. They had read the account of the St. Louis tooth discovery in the newspapers, and were impressed. But something had bothered them. Barry Commoner, the former Washington University biology professor who led the original study, was skeptical about the possibility to evaluate health risks from Strontium-90 in old baby teeth. "To use this for an epidemiological link is very iffy," said Commoner, who was still active professionally in his mid-80s. "They mean well, but I have never associated myself with their results."

These comments were strange, given that Commoner had suggested the teeth be given to RPHP. Moreover, years ago he had argued strenuously for a study evaluating childhood cancer risk from bomb fallout by studying Sr-90 in teeth, only to be told by Harold Rosenthal that such a study was not possible with the lab instruments then available. Nobody at RPHP had any explanation for Commoner's thoughts. Soon after the phone call, Deer Creek rejected the RPHP proposal. Several other applications followed in St. Louis and elsewhere, but all were rejected. The prevailing reason was that such a study had little relevance – bomb testing above the ground had ended with the 1963 Treaty.

But in truth, the issue is a current one still unresolved decades later. About 140 million Americans exposed to bomb fallout are still alive. Virtually all of them have a family member or friend who has suffered from cancer, and many still don't know the cause.

The U.S. government insisted that bomb fallout hadn't harmed one single

American until 1997, when the National Cancer Institute issued a report. (The report had begun 15 years before, and had been completed 5 years earlier, only to sit on the desk of the U.S. Energy Secretary). The massive, 100,000 page study, whose release was forced by Energy Department official Robert Alvarez, made estimates of Iodine-131 exposures from Nevada bomb tests in the 1950s and 1960s for all Americans, according to their place of residence, birth date, gender, and milk drinking habits.

The findings were shocking. The doses from iodine-131 were more than 100 times greater than government estimates years earlier. Some counties in Idaho and Montana received hundreds of times more exposure than in less-hard hit areas, such as much of the west coast and desert southwest. The estimate from the report was that between 11,000 and 212,000 Americans developed thyroid cancer just from I-131 exposure from the Nevada tests. The report was a landmark, but it did not cover the dozens of other radioactive chemicals, nor did it examine harm from U.S. tests in the Pacific, and Soviet tests in Siberia.

Some hoped that the 1997 study would be a springboard for more analyses – but exactly the opposite happened. The following year, an expert panel at the Institute of Medicine reported that there is no good way to identify just which Americans developed cancer from bomb tests. The panel also sought to soften the 1997 study by stating that the number of thyroid cancer cases caused by fallout was probably at the low end of the National Cancer Institute estimate, and that thyroid cancer was rarely fatal. "Tell that to my brother," shot back U.S. Senator Tom Harkin, whose brother had died of the disease.

The U.S. Department of Health and Human Services released a study in 2003 concluding that at least 11,000 cancer deaths were caused by bomb fallout in the past half century. This was a tiny number, considering that tens of million Americans were exposed to fallout, including the susceptible Baby Boomers born during the bomb test era, when fallout from American and Soviet explosions amounted to 40,000 Hiroshima bombs.

The final blow came in 2005, when federal funding was terminated for a study of effects of bomb fallout being done by Dr. Joseph Lyon of the University of Utah. Even long after the Cold War had ended, the U.S. government had cut and run on the issue of health effects of bomb test fallout. The answer to the question of what fallout – both from weapons tests and reactors operations - had done to Americans is largely an emphatic "nobody knows."

The St. Louis baby teeth offer a good chance to answer that question. There is probably no other way quite as accurate to identify the buildup of fallout in American bodies. Certainly, there is no other sample of similar size. And with nearly four decades having passed since the study ended, and with the ability to find death records of deceased tooth donors and health histories of living ones, now is an ideal time to make such a study.

The flurry of recent events surrounding the discovery of St. Louis baby teeth extends a journey that has lasted half a century. Scientists and citizens alike have wanted to understand how much man made radioactivity – from nuclear weapons and reactors – have entered human bodies, and to understand how it has harmed health. Much has been accomplished, but there is a long way to go. The story of the quest for this knowledge is related in this book.

CHAPTER 2
CANCER VICTIMS SEEK CAUSE, NOT JUST CURE

Agnes Reynolds stared at her son Jon. The pre-teen was playing in their backyard just outside Hartford CT, ignoring Agnes' repeated calls that dinner was ready. As she had done many times in the past few years, Agnes' thoughts drifted away from dinner to what had happened to Jon.

In late 1991, Agnes and her husband Gilbert were delighted to finally become parents. And lo and behold, healthy twin babies Jon and Michelle were presented to the world. Parenting twins was no easy task, as Agnes found out, as it took all of her energy to take care of them. Even though she was used to working long and intensive hours as a nurse, this was much more exhausting. But it was also much more gratifying.

Her thoughts went back to Easter 1996. Jon had vomited after dinner, and was irritable and pale. She was concerned, but not worried that it may have been more than a stomach bug. But the problems didn't go away. Fevers, nausea and vomiting continued. The Reynolds' doctor examined the boy, and suggested further testing, and Agnes now knew it was serious.

The oncologist gave the shocking, but not surprising diagnosis of leukemia, a cancer of the blood organs. Jon was given chemotherapy right away, beginning a three-year ordeal in which the treatment feels just as bad as the disease. Luckily, the cancer went into remission almost immediately. After the treatment ended, Jon was able to lead a normal life and is now an energetic teenager. But because he and his family know the disease could return at any time, periodic tests are done to check it.

As the chemo ended and Jon returned to health, Agnes found herself asking questions. Why did this happen? Why Jon? Why now? She could think of no obvious risk factor that would make her son more likely to develop leukemia. She began to pose questions to her doctors, but still nothing emerged. She began poring through the internet, and found that little was known about what causes children to develop cancer.

She did find many theories on causation, the most common of these being exposure to radiation. This was based on the premise that fetuses, infants, and children are most vulnerable to radiation, something she knew from her nursing career. She found out that for many years, doctors would give pregnant women X-rays to their abdomen, for routine purposes, like understanding how large the child was and how it was positioned in the womb. After studies showing that children whose mother had been given an X-ray before birth were much more likely to develop cancer during childhood, the practice stopped and was replaced by ultrasound (which emits no radiation).

In her travels from web site to web site, Agnes came upon a group called the Radiation and Public Health Project (RPHP). This was a group of health researchers that was examining the link between radiation exposure and cancer – especially in children. Interesting, she thought. She discovered that the group was collecting baby teeth and testing them for radiation levels. Moreover, the group was interested in donations of teeth from children who have cancer. Agnes reached for the telephone and dialed the group's number.

Jane Furst was not somebody who easily believed that miracles could happen. She was a trained and experienced nurse, married to a financial professional, and a practical mother of two young boys. When it came to health, she believed what she had been taught and practiced good health habits. No smoking. No excessive drinking. Good diet. Adequate exercise. Periodic visits to the doctor for checkups, for her and her sons.

But in a short period in January 1992, Jane found herself grasping for a miracle. Her younger son Cory didn't feel quite right to her. "His abdomen felt hard, unusually hard," she recalls. Only two days later, she and her husband Joel stood in the emergency room of a hospital near their New Jersey home, staring at a CAT scan and hearing the unbelievable news, that their baby, just 19 months old, had cancer.

The disease was in Cory's liver and lung, and so large and advanced that doctors were forced to immediately administer chemotherapy to shrink the tumor, then do surgery to remove more tissue. The chances were not great that he would pull through, said the doctors. It would take kind of a miracle.

The chemotherapy proved to be a brutal experience for Cory, who was constantly in pain, weak, nauseous, and lethargic. For three months, Jane stayed round the clock at the hospital with her son, unable to leave his side. The tumors shrank, the surgery was successful, and after four more rounds of chemotherapy, the cancer was in remission and Cory was sent home. Cory is now an energetic high school student, with no apparent signs of ever having been sick other than that his hearing is impaired and that he cannot play vigorous sports. The eight-month ordeal had ended in a miracle

During the nightmarish days of 1992, Jane had to maintain a focus on Cory's treatment. But once the cancer receded and Cory resumed his life, she began to wonder. "We never did anything wrong," she thought, remembering that she and Joel were healthy human beings with terrific health habits. Jane showed her gratitude to the network of hospitals and doctors who had pulled Cory through, by volunteering her time with various childhood cancer programs.

One of these programs was the Tomorrow Children's Fund, which was based at the Hackensack University Medical Center in Hackensack NJ. One day Jane received a letter from Deirdre Imus, who ran an Environmental Center for Pediatric Oncology out of the hospital. Deirdre was a young woman married to radio personality Don Imus, who had long been associated with the Tomorrow Children's Fund. The letter, sent to each member of the Fund, described a study that was measuring radiation in baby teeth, and asked each child to donate a tooth.

Jane had never heard of the study, or of the group conducting it, called the Radiation and Public Health Project. But before long, she was watching Cory speak at a press conference at Hackensack, where New Jersey Governor James McGreevey announced that $25,000 from the state legislature would be given to RPHP to cover costs of the study. As Cory held up his tooth for reporters to see, Jane realized that her desire for a miracle was now accompanied by a desire for a cause.

While cancer is all too common in America, it is relatively rare in children. Until the mid 1900s, it was almost an oddity. Few pediatric oncologists (doctors who specialize in childhood cancer) existed, and few pediatricians could detect symptoms of cancer in children. Few treatments existed, so most children stricken with the disease died.

The effort to help children with cancer was given a boost in the years following World War II, in which greater federal funding for hospitals and medical research helped scientists develop new treatments, including cancer treatments. Another reason may have been the large jump in childhood cancer rates. From 1937 to 1950, the number of American children under age ten that died from cancer jumped from 1361 to 2778, which translates to a 53% increase in the death rate. Half of these deaths were from leukemia.

But in the second half of the 20th century, there was a remarkable improvement in child cancer therapy. These included surgical techniques, chemotherapy, and radiation therapy (some types of radiation help treat cancer, as it kills cancerous cells). Many more children survived cancer, and lived into adulthood. Today, the child death rate is only about one-third what it was in 1950.

Even though the treatments are keeping more children alive, the reality is not that sunny. Treatments are often grueling ordeals that last months and even years, with many side effects. Survivors have been found to be more likely to develop other physical problems. They are more likely to have developmental problems, and complete fewer years of school than other children. And of course, the fear that the cancer will some day return is something the child and their loved ones must live with for the rest of their lives. Currently, about 250,000 Americans, adults and children, are survivors of childhood cancer.

In addition, the cost of treating children with cancer is becoming prohibitive, and cutbacks in health insurance makes treatment less affordable with time. In 2003, a newspaper article revealed that the prestigious Columbia Presbyterian Medical Center in New York City was facing a half-million dollar deficit with its child cancer program, and was likely to cut physicians, nurses, and other staff to balance the budget.

Unlike cancer death rates, cancer incidence rates, or rates of diagnosed cases, have not dropped in recent years. Connecticut developed a statewide cancer registry for all cases in 1935, years before any other state did. Compared to the late 1930s, the rate of childhood cancer is nearly twice as high today. Some claim that the rise is mostly due to better methods of diagnosing cases. But most believe the increase is a real one. About 13,000 American children age 19 or under receive a diagnosis of cancer each year.

In the lengthy effort to better treat childhood cancer, much less attention has been paid to understand what causes the disease. Funds to understand causes have been limited, and research is usually conducted by health professionals at universities on their own time. The reasons why children develop cancer are much different than those for adults. Personal habits, such as smoking, eating certain foods, and alcohol consumption are not factors for children, making the understanding of cause more difficult.

But for a long time, scientists have understood that various types of radiation exposure have caused cancer in humans, especially in children, for two reasons. First, any type of radiation kills or damages cells in the human body. Because the fetus, infant, and child is growing so quickly, its cells are dividing at a rapid rate. A damaged cell in a small human will duplicate (into other damaged cells) much faster, which could lead to cancer. Second, when a person is exposed to radiation and cells are damaged, the body's immune system tries to repair any damage. The fetal, infant, and child immune system is still not well developed, and thus is less likely to return the cells to healthy ones.

For years, medical doctors have been aware of the risks to children from X-rays. Dentists typically will not take X-rays of young children because of the health risks involved, even though X-ray machines yield lower doses of radiation than they did years ago. Doctors try not to give CAT scans to children unless they are absolutely necessary.

Sometimes scientists have learned about cancer risk to children from radiation exposure the hard way. In the 1950s, British physician Alice Stewart found that when pregnant women received an X-ray to the abdomen, the risk that the baby would die from cancer before age ten doubled. At the time, doctors performed these diagnostic X-rays on thousands of women, thinking that the dose from the X-ray was so low that no harm could be possible. Naturally, Stewart's studies caused a howl from obstetricians, radiologists, and other scientists. Her work was dismissed by many. But follow-up studies by Stewart and others confirmed that even this low dose caused childhood cancer. The practice of abdominal X-rays before birth was halted in the 1970s.

While X-rays were first used about 1900, another type of radiation was introduced nearly 50 years later. This was fission. Scientists found that when uranium atoms were split in a laboratory, it caused very high energy to be produced. The splitting process was known as fission. Refining of the fission process led to the development of the world's first atomic bombs. The United States dropped bombs on the Japanese cities of Hiroshima and Nagasaki, causing tremendous devastation and ending World War II.

The atomic bomb introduced to the world new chemicals that emitted ionizing radiation, so named because splitting uranium atoms caused electrons (or ions) to break off and to create unstable, radioactive chemicals. The fission process created over 100 chemicals, many of which did not exist in nature. These chemicals included Cesium-137, Iodine-131, Plutonium-239, and Strontium-90.

Although atomic bombs were never used on people after 1945, many bombs were exploded as tests in unpopulated areas. The U.S. tested 206 bombs above the ground in the Marshall Islands and at the Nevada Test Site, about 70 miles north of Las Vegas, from 1946 to 1962. American tests yielded the equivalent of 10,000 Hiroshima bombs of radioactivity, while Soviet tests yielded an additional 30,000 Hiroshima bombs.

Each of these tests created large mushroom clouds filled with the 100-plus fission products. Some of the chemicals quickly fell to the ground near the test site. But much of the cloud soared high into the stratosphere and moved with the prevailing winds. Because winds generally blow from the west to the east fallout spread across the continental United States. The fallout stayed in the stratosphere until rain and snow brought it down to the earth - and into people's bodies. Some of it was breathed. Some of it was consumed in water, as it reached reservoirs or private wells. Some of it was consumed in milk (after contaminated grass was eaten by cows). And some of it was consumed in vegetables, fish, and meat.

Each radioactive chemical in the fallout clouds decays over time. Some chemicals decay quickly, while others last much longer. The decay rate is measured as a half-life, or the amount of time it takes for a chemical to decay to half its original quantity. Some of these chemicals are listed below. Because chemicals such as Plutonium-239 have such a long half life, they essentially stay in the environment forever.

Short Half-Life		Long Half-Life	
Strontium-89	50.5 days	Strontium-90	(28.7 years)
Iodine-131	8.0 days	Iodine-129	(15.7 million years)
Cesium-134	2.0 days	Cesium-137	(30.0 years)
Xenon-133	5.3 days	Plutonium-239	(24,400 years)

Nuclear weapons tests above the ground continued until 1963, when a treaty banning such tests became law (this will be discussed later in more detail). Thereafter, testing continued at below-ground sites; the U.S. conducted over 900 such tests at the Nevada site. These tests released the same radioactive chemical mix, but it was much better contained, and much less of it entered human bodies than from above-ground tests. Since 1992, virtually no atomic weapons tests have been conducted worldwide.

The mixture of fission products is found in other sources in addition to nuclear weapons, mostly in nuclear reactors. The earliest reactors were for the purpose of building bombs, and later reactors produced electricity. Much of the radioactivity was contained in reactor buildings; because the mix of chemicals is dangerous and because it serves no purpose after creating weapons and electricity, it must be stored as nuclear waste. An enormous amount of this waste now exists at many U.S. nuclear plants.

But some of the radioactivity escapes into the air, despite the best efforts of reactor operators to contain it. And just like it did after bomb tests, it was breathed, eaten, and drank by humans. And although bomb testing went underground years ago and later stopped altogether, nuclear reactors are still operating. Since 1998, the total of U.S. reactors that produce electricity has held steady at 104, located at 65 nuclear plants (some plants have more than one reactor). All nuclear weapons plants had stopped operating by 1991.

For the past half century, the debate over whether these chemicals have caused cancer, especially in children, has raged. It has been a political debate, not just a scientific one. The bomb testing program was done to build up the American military arsenal, at a time when many believed that a nuclear war with the Soviet Union was inevitable. The nuclear reactors were a multibillion dollar business run by private utility companies. With the stakes so high, it was inevitable that the radiation health issue would be controversial.

The controversy was made worse by the limits of research. How can a researcher prove, beyond the shadow of a doubt, that radiation causes cancer? The answer: it's not easy. Many factors can affect whether someone develops cancer. A heavy smoker who develops lung cancer was certainly harmed by cigarettes – but genetics, chemicals breathed on the job and in the environment, and other factors may have played a role. With the bar set so high to prove cause, controversy was inevitable.

But researchers do have plenty of tools to show that an environmental poison such as radiation caused cancer. Even before the era of nuclear weapons and reactors, scientists had found childhood cancer to be caused by exposure. Experiments on animals showed that radiation was especially harmful to the young. In addition, studies of infants who received X-rays to treat diseases showed that they were much more likely to develop cancer as children. Stewart's research with diagnostic X-rays showed that even a low dose of radiation harms infants and children.

The United States has a republican form of government. In theory, if the majority supports a certain policy, the nation's leaders will also support it. Moreover, the nation is also a democracy. Citizens have the ability to become directly involved in policy matters, and thus can affect these policies. In the quest to understand if there is a link between childhood cancer and radiation exposure, there can be considerable input from the people, not just the scientific elite.

So late in the 20th century, several factors converged:

- The rising number of children with cancer in their body
- The politics of nuclear weapons
- The politics of nuclear reactors
- The limits of scientific research to prove cause
- The ability of citizens to affect research policies

With these in place, on a course to all come together, the story of studies of radiation in baby teeth can be told.

CHAPTER 3
COLD WAR BRINGS CITIZENS AND SCIENTISTS TOGETHER

After World War II ended, the world entered a much-needed cooling off period after years of devastation. In America, millions of troops came home and picked up their pre-war lives. The draft was terminated. President Harry S. Truman, who had ordered the atom bombs dropped on Japan, kept America's nuclear program, but at a relatively slow pace. In the first five years after the war, just five nuclear weapons were tested in the south Pacific. With the Germans and Japanese defeated, no hostile nation threatened the U.S.

But the pause was a short one, as another threat emerged. This time it was Communism. During the year from mid-1949 to mid-1950, several developments thrust the U.S. into a new kind of war, called the Cold War. Communist forces led by Mao Tse-Tung overran China. Communist troops from North Korea invaded the south, and the U.S. entered the Korean War. Maybe the most shocking of the new developments was the announcement that the Soviet Union had successfully exploded their own atomic bomb – using technology stolen from the American program.

With an openly aggressive regime led by Joseph Stalin in Moscow, Truman made several decisions. One of these was to test more bombs, and test them closer to home. Several sites were considered, and the Nevada Test Site selected. The site was actually on a piece of government-owned land already used as a bombing and gunnery range. It was a bleak, desolate stretch of desert, with only small numbers of wild animals across the desert signifying that life existed there. Truman's staff selected it because it was unpopulated, and because the wind blew toward the east, away from the populated California coast.

The first test in Nevada took place at 5:44 on the morning of January 27, 1951, a blast given the code name of Able. Although government officials were pleased with their selection of the Nevada site, what they saw after Able was shocking. The towering fallout cloud, which was 300 miles in width, began moving rapidly across the nation to the east. By the afternoon of the 27th, it was over St. Louis, about 1400 miles from the blast. On the morning of the 29th, a snowstorm over the northeast brought down the fallout, and scientists reported that their Geiger counters were clicking wildly. Four more blasts in Nevada followed Able over the next ten days, and the nuclear arms race had officially started.

During the rest of the 1950s, the United States made an all-out effort to develop a mighty arsenal of nuclear weapons, and testing went on furiously. By 1958, the U.S. had tested 206 bombs, virtually all of them above the ground, and many more than the Soviet total of 53 and the British total of 21. Government leaders, starting with President Dwight D. Eisenhower, proclaimed the program to be a success, citing the need for nuclear superiority.

The reaction of Americans to the bomb testing was a mixed one. At first, people were relatively quiet. The newness of the program and the awesome spectacle of shot after shot – they were all pre-announced and many were televised – was a lot to take in. Moreover, a culture of trust in government was a strong one. The government, and especially the military, was held in high esteem. After all, it had led the country to victory in a world war. Military leaders such as Eisenhower and Douglas MacArthur were national heroes. If government leaders said that bomb tests were necessary to counter the Soviet threat, it was true in the minds of most. And if government leaders said the program was carried out safely, it was also true.

Stories of people living closest to the tests, in southern Utah are most amazing. Many people, even hundreds of miles away, could see the blasts with the naked eye. Those who lived closest could hear the roar that accompanied each test, and even felt the rumblings in the earth. But the citizens simply carried on. The love of country and fear of Communism was too dominant, and had no room for questions of safety. One resident recalled later

> "The big pink cloud that hung over us for more than a day…we walked in it, breathed it, washed our clothes in it, hung our clothes out in it – very few people had driers in those times and even the little children ate the snow. You know the little kids love snow. They went out and would eat the snow. They didn't know it was going to kill them later on."

Media reports went along with the government program as well. The military invited the press to film and report on various blasts. Stories generally were descriptive of the explosions and fallout clouds that followed. Reports from Utah, a state with a large majority of conservative Mormons, were virtually all positive, even though it was receiving the most fallout of any state.

But an undercurrent of worry took hold of many people, not just in Utah but all across America. Government officials took immediate action. In 1950, as Communism and nuclear weapons became issues, the federal Civil Defense Administration made a nine-minute animated black-and-white film aimed at schoolchildren called "Duck and Cover." A character called Bert the Turtle cheerfully informed kids of what to do in case of a nuclear attack. They would simply have to "duck and cover" – or get under their desks face down, curl up into a fetal position, and cover their heads with their hands, so that any flying objects hurled from the powerful blast would not hurt their heads. A female chorus sang the jingle as the words "duck and cover" came across the screen.

This film was shown in many classrooms throughout the 1950s and 1960s. Years later, Baby Boom children remember the film with laughter, as they know that nuclear weapons can easily destroy society, and ducking-and-covering can do nothing to stop fallout from entering the air, food, and water. One Boomer recalled:

> "I used to have nightmares about the 'Bomb' when I was a kid. It was such a nebulous but terrifying thing. In school we had this sort of 'duck and cover' propaganda complete with drills and explanations about the 'bright flash' etc. Come on, we were little kids, what did they think we were going to think? Obviously, they didn't think of that. Case in point: As a child, one of my big fears was that this horrible thing called the 'Bomb' would happen WHEN I WAS NOT AT SCHOOL! To my 6-year old mind, the only safe place in the world was under my desk at school!"

But despite the attempts of government to calm people, unquestioned trust gave way to anxious suspicion and questions. The first of these questions were raised, ironically, in Utah. In the afternoon of March 24, 1953, the test shot named Nancy exploded over the Nevada desert. The bomb had a yield of 24 kilotons, making it one of the largest to date. The fallout moved across the country, but not before it first deposited significant amounts of radioactivity in southeastern Utah.

The closest population to the test site was in the two Utah counties, Iron and Washington (the part of Nevada east of the test site had virtually no residents). First inhabited by the Paiute Indians and colonized by the Spanish, Mormons had begun to settle the area in the 1850s. By the time of the bomb testing, about 20,000 persons lived in the two counties. Because of the warm climate and the rugged mountains, agriculture (mostly sheep herding) became the economic mainstay of the region.

In the spring of 1953, soon after the Nancy shot, sheep and lambs began to suddenly die on their grazing areas. The toll within a few weeks reached over 4,000, and many exhibited burns on their skin so typical of radiation poisoning. For the first time, local farmers questioned whether bomb fallout was harming their communities. Naturally, officials from the Atomic Energy Commission investigated. They found many sheep had thyroid glands that were destroyed, and high levels of radioactive Iodine-131 which is so harmful to this organ. Gastrointestinal tracts of sheep also had very high radiation levels.

But the AEC kept these findings secret. At public hearings, it blatantly denied that any unusual burns had been found on sheep, and in its official report, it concluded instead that the sheep had died of malnutrition. Local citizens were now alarmed, to the point that they filed a law suit against the AEC which would spend decades in the courts. The bubble of trust in the bomb testing program had been burst.

Various stories began to emerge from citizens living in the small towns in southwestern Utah. Mrs. Frankie Bentley of the town of Parowan recalled

> "In 1960 we had four young teenagers die with leukemia, first ever in the Parowan area...We have just a personal suffering of a small community for we are all involved with each others lives. The damage is done with us and it will be for a long time."

As people began raising questions, the media publicized them. Newspapers began to publish reports on where in the United States the fallout was penetrating, and sometimes publicized levels in the air and milk. Politicians also began to ask questions, the most outspoken of which was Adlai Stevenson. In 1956, Stevenson was the Democratic nominee for President. Trailing badly to the popular Eisenhower, Stevenson seized on the nuclear issue as a way to distance himself from Eisenhower. Stevenson spoke out against testing hydrogen bombs (a more powerful type of nuclear weapon that had been developed), citing the hazards from fallout. The speech summed up what many Americans now believed:

"With every explosion of a super-bomb huge quantities off radioactive materials are thrown up into the air – pumped into the air currents of the world at all altitudes – and later on they fall to earth as dust or in rain.

I don't wish to be an alarmist and I'm not asserting that the present levels of radioactivity are dangerous. Scientists don't know exactly how dangerous the threat is, but they do know that the threat will increase if we go on testing."

Stevenson had given the fallout issue a national forum for the first time. Now that Americans were catching on to the threat of fallout, there were questions to be answered. How much fallout was getting into the environment? How much was actually entering people's bodies? And was fallout harming people, especially our young?

In the mid-1950s, research on health effects of radiation from atomic bombs was virtually unheard of. The first reports were coming in about the survivors of the Hiroshima and Nagasaki blasts. In just several years, they were developing cancer at higher-than-expected rates. In fact, the leukemia rate for all of Japan rose 50% from 1946 to the early 1950s. But there was nothing else.

During the early years of the American bomb tests, there was no system to measure how much radioactivity was getting into the air, water, and food. Sporadic measurements by scientists showed a rise in environmental levels, but as the tests went on, a better system was needed. Local health departments lacked the equipment and expertise to make these measurements. This was a problem for the federal government.

The 1956 presidential campaign, the buildup of fallout, and pressure applied by citizens caused the Eisenhower administration to create a system of measuring bomb test fallout in the environment. The following spring, the U.S. Public Health Service system began, covering five U.S. cities, which rose to nine in 1958 and 60 in 1960. Air, water, and milk samples were included in the monthly reports.

Of particular interest was the milk samples, since infants and children need to drink plenty of milk to aid in growth. Iodine-131, Barium-140, Strontium-89, Strontium-90, Cesium-137, radioactive calcium, and radioactive potassium were measured, and results were astonishing. The fast-decaying radioactive chemicals soared in the months of testing and returned to zero within a month or two. Levels of slow-decaying chemicals moved gradually higher.

Of the nine cities in the initial Public Health Service program, the highest levels were in St. Louis, followed by Atlanta. Even though Salt Lake City was closest to the test site, it receives much less rain than the cities in the Midwest and Southeast, and thus had less radioactivity in milk. The lowest levels were in the very dry Austin Texas, and in Sacramento California, which was located west (upwind) of the Nevada Test Site. The average levels of Strontium-90 in milk for August-December 1958, the first months in which measurements were made for all nine sites, illustrate these great variations (given in picocuries of Strontium-90 per liter of raw milk.

Site	Sr-90
St. Louis	15.48
Atlanta	11.02
Cincinnati	10.06
Spokane	8.84
Chicago	7.72
New York City	7.02
Salt Lake City	4.72
Sacramento	4.46
Austin	3.74

While the Public Health Service dutifully continued to collect data, it did little else. Published volumes were not widely circulated or publicized. More importantly, the measurements were always accompanied by the government's assurance that levels were much too low to cause any harm to humans – even though they had not done any actual research on the subject, and were not funding any such research. But many people refused to believe the government. They knew fallout levels in the diet were rising, and they were not satisfied.

The program to measure how much fallout was getting into the bodies of Americans had a slow start as well. Scientists were not sure if low dose radiation could be detected using the equipment available at that time. But in July 1953, just two years after the bomb testing began in Nevada, scientists attending a conference at the Rand Corporation in California showed that testing was able to accurately detect fallout levels in animals. The scientists agreed to initiate a world wide program measuring fallout in humans. They also agreed that they would focus on Strontium-90 in human bones.

Strontium is a metal that is similar to calcium, first discovered in the 1700s. There are non-radioactive forms of Strontium that have existed in nature for many thousands of years. The chemical is not as well known as hydrogen, oxygen, and calcium. But this all changed in the 1940s, when the splitting of uranium atoms created several new forms of Strontium – radioactive forms. Strontium-89 and Strontium-87 have short half lives and decay quickly. But Strontium-90 is another story.

Sr-90 has a physical half life of 28.7 years, which means outside the body, like in milk, water, and shed baby teeth, it decays until half of its original amount remains after 28.7 years. Sr-90, like all types of Strontium, is similar to calcium. When it enters the body through breathing and the food chain, the body thinks it is calcium. Quickly after reaching the stomach, Sr-90 moves to the bloodstream and then attaches to bone and teeth. Some of it leaves the body through the urine.

Any radioactive chemical can be seen as a wild bull in a china shop. Unlike most chemicals it is unstable, and smashes into cells, breaking membrane on the outside of the cell and hitting the nucleus inside the cell. The damage done to cells can sometimes kill the cell entirely. If the cell does not die, it can repair the damage – or not. A damaged cell will reproduce into more damaged cells, raising the chance the cell will mutate and cancer will develop.

Sr-90 gives off harmful beta particles once in the cell. It damages teeth and bone, and the beta particles can penetrate into the bone marrow. When it decays, it is replaced by a "daughter product", a chemical known as Yttrium-90. Y-90 is also radioactive, and enters the pituitary gland at the base of the throat.

As mentioned, Sr-90 is only one of over 100 chemicals formed when atomic bombs explode and nuclear reactors operate. Each represents a health risk, as each is radioactive and each can cause cancer. Some enter organs much more sensitive than the bone and teeth, such as the lung. Some are emitted in much greater quantities than Sr-90. Some last much longer than Sr-90; for example, plutonium-239 has a half life of 24,400 years.

But from the early years of bomb testing, it was Sr-90 more than any other chemical that drew the most concern from scientists and the public, for several reasons. Sr-90 decays relatively slowly, and remains in the environment and body longer than most radioactive chemicals. About half of the Sr-90 in the diet is from drinking milk, the most crucial food in the development of the young.

But perhaps the biggest reason for the worry caused by Sr-90 was its ability to penetrate into the bone marrow. It is in the marrow that the white blood cells are formed, the same white blood cells that form the basis for the immune system's defenses. If these cells are damaged by Sr-90, the body cannot properly heal itself. So Sr-90 is a risk factor not just for bone cancer, but for all cancers, and other immune-related diseases including asthma, allergies, ear infections, and even the common cold.

The federal government assigned a group of researchers from Columbia University in New York the task of finding out how much fallout was building up in human bodies, not just in the United States, but around the world. Knowing that Sr-90 was detectable in low levels in animal bones, the Columbia team began collecting rib bones from deceased persons. The initial network involved 16 locations, including four U.S. cities and Puerto Rico. Rib bones were analyzed in a special laboratory run by experts in measuring radioactive chemicals.

By late 1956, the group had tested over 500 bones, and published an article in the journal Science. The findings confirmed exactly what they had suspected:

- Sr-90 had entered the bodies of people all around the world

- North America, which received the bulk of the fallout from tests in Nevada and the Pacific, had higher levels of Sr-90 than Europe and South America

- Infants and children had much higher levels of Sr-90 than did adults

- As the testing went on, levels of Sr-90 in bone became higher and higher

The group, concerned about the buildup of fallout in bodies, continued to collect bone samples, and published several articles through the 1960s. But throughout their work, the Columbia team insisted that the amount of Sr-90 in bones were well below "permissible limits," about 1% or less than such limits, and thus did not present a health risk to humans, a mantra repeated over and over by government officials.

Except for these articles, the government bone project was kept relatively secret. But years later in the 1990s, it was revealed that this secrecy also meant a gross lack of ethics. The Atomic Energy Commission failed to request permission from the next of kin of the deceased, and cut their bodies and removed bones that they then analyzed for Sr-90. Transcripts of meetings showed that researchers were well aware of the ethical and legal violations they were making, but were more concerned about getting enough bones to make their studies significant. In 1955, AEC Commissioner and University of Chicago researcher Willard Libby commented on the bone samples:

> "I don't know how to get them, but I do say that it is a matter of prime importance to get them and particularly in the young age group. So, human samples are of prime importance, and if anybody knows how to a good job of body snatching, they will be really be serving their country."

Just before the article on the AEC bone program went to press, Adlai Stevenson gave his campaign speech calling for a testing halt. Part of Stevenson's speech was about the hazards of fallout, and he specifically singled out Sr-90 as especially poisonous. The term that just recently was known only to a handful of scientists now had become a household word.

> "This radioactive fall-out as it is called, carries something that's called strontium-90, which is the most dreadful poison in the world. For only one tablespoon equally shared by all the members of the human race could produce a dangerous level of radioactivity in the bones of every individual. In sufficient concentrations it can cause bone cancer and dangerously affect the reproductive processes."

Stevenson wouldn't say whether enough Sr-90 had been consumed to harm people. But others went further than Stevenson. University of Rochester biochemist William Neuman who was an expert on radiation in bone stated that instead of under 1 percent of permissible limits, American children would accumulate 10 percent of these limits in their bones. If testing continued, the levels would go higher. Neuman also scotched the notion of a "permissible limit" of radiation, because of the difficulty in estimating such a limit.

Dr. Evarts Graham of the Washington University School of Medicine in St. Louis wrote Stevenson a letter in the fall of 1956, asserting

> "Scientific facts known to the Eisenhower administration disprove the administration's official stand that danger to human life from radioactive strontium 90 fallout is 'negligible'… present strontium 90 levels are a public health problem of serious magnitude."

Even as Stevenson lost the election, the Sr-90 issue did not disappear from the radar screen of the American public. On the contrary, the concerns grew, and politicians began to respond to the majority. Senator Hubert Humphrey informed farmers that Sr-90 concentration in Wisconsin and Illinois soil had quadrupled in the past two years. Governor Averill Harriman reported that Sr-90 levels in New York state were 10 to 60 times higher than normal, a claim later backed up by figures in the environment and human bodies.

Fear over nuclear weapons picked up even more in 1957. That year, the greatest radioactivity in Nevada bomb tests was released. In July, the largest single test in Nevada, named Hood, took place, with the explosive power of five Hiroshima bombs. The following month came the Smoky shot. It too was much more powerful than Hiroshima, but this was also one of the blasts in which military personnel were sent close to the test site soon after the blast to simulate the "takeover" of a nuclear weapon target.

About 250 soldiers moved within 100 yards just minutes after the explosion. But the shot had gone very wrong; scientists miscalculated the power of the blast, and the direction of the wind. The soldiers were in a "hot spot" and had to be evacuated in a hurry, but not after being exposed to high doses of radiation. One of the soldiers recalled

> "The heat was so intense, I felt as though my uniform was going to catch on fire… Scientists who approached from a different direction had to abandon their attempt to retrieve instruments because of intense radioactivity. The instruments were left in the field for several days until the radiation disappeared."

Years later, an unusually large number of these soldiers developed cancer, and went through an extensive legal process to be compensated for the harm they received. After Smoky, fallout in the American diet reached an all time high.

Another 1957 event that galvanized Americans about nuclear weapons was the publication of Nevil Shute's book On the Beach. Shute, a British novelist, had served in both world wars and was concerned about the potential for another, much more devastating war with nuclear weapons. The book takes place just after a series of nuclear weapons destroyed life on earth except in Australia, and details the last desperate days of several people living in that nation watching radioactive fallout move steadily towards them before they too are poisoned and die. The book became a best seller, and made into a movie in 1959 starring Gregory Peck and Ava Gardner.

In 1957, scientists also stood up for a halt to testing as never before. Several world-recognized scientists spoke out strongly against nuclear war and fallout. One was Dr. Albert Schweitzer, a physician and Nobel Peace Prize winner best known for his work to establish hospitals and clinics in impoverished areas of Africa. In April, the 82-year old Schweitzer broadcast a "Declaration of Conscience" from Norway, spelling out his desire for an end to bomb testing and his concerns about nuclear fallout:

> "The material (on fallout) collected, although far from complete, allows us to draw the conclusion that radiation resulting from the explosions which have already taken place represents a danger to the human race – a danger not to be underrated – and that further explosions of atomic bombs will increase this danger to an alarming extent."

Schweitzer mentioned Strontium-90 as being "particularly dangerous" and "present in large amounts in the radioactive dust." He also warned that children are at particular risk:

> "To the profound damage of these cells corresponds a profound damage to our descendents. It consists in stillbirths and in the births of babies with mental or physical defects."

He warned about the dangers to not just living humans but their descendents, and also cautioned that "even the weakest of internal radiation can have harmful effects on our descendents" putting him at odds with government officials who continued to preach that exposures below permissible limits were harmless.

The other world-renowned scientist who took a stand in 1957 was Linus Pauling. Like Schweitzer, Pauling was a Nobel Prize winner who had never become actively involved in a political issue before. In May Pauling wrote the Scientists Bomb Test Appeal calling for an end to testing, and worked to obtain the signatures of over 9,000 scientists. Pauling delivered the petition to the United Nations on January 15, 1958. When he won a Nobel Peace prize several years later, he issued a warning about fallout's damage to children, stating that bomb fallout would cause genetic damage "such as to lead to an increase in the number of seriously defective children that will be born in future generations."

The work of Pauling and others finally forced the hands of American and Soviet leaders. In the fall of 1958, each nation agreed to observe a moratorium on bomb testing. It was progress, but represented only a temporary halt in a fragile co-existence between the two nations that possessed the power to destroy life on the planet.

With both citizens and scientists concerned about the fallout problem, it made sense that the two groups should combine forces. The melding of scientists and citizens became a reality in St. Louis. A number of faculty members at Washington University had already spoken publicly against the continuation of testing. These included physicist John Fowler, pathologist Walter Bauer, and biologist Barry Commoner. Early in 1958, they decided that a group of scientists and citizens was needed to collect and present information on fallout to the public.

The three professors approached Edna Gellhorn, a prominent St. Louis public figure who had been president of the local League of Women Voters. A March 23, 1958 meeting produced the following statement, and the Greater St. Louis Citizen's Committee for Nuclear Information was born:

> "We resolve to establish the Greater St. Louis Citizen's Committee for Nuclear Information to collect and distribute information about the consequences of nuclear weapons tests, nuclear warfare, and other uses of nuclear energy, in order that the public may become sufficiently informed to contribute effectively to the development of

sound public policies on these vital issues."

A steering committee was named, and the group went about the business of organizing its goals and recruiting members.

CHAPTER 4
ST. LOUIS TOOTH STUDY OF BOMB TEST FALLOUT – EARLY YEARS

The Committee wasted no time in bringing the bomb testing issue to the public's attention. It quickly started a newsletter, entitled Nuclear Information, and circulated it. It made a strong effort to increase membership, which reached 400 by the end of 1958. It established a speakers' bureau of scientific experts, and began to make public presentations on various nuclear-related topics.

The risk to health, especially children's health, was a standard message presented by the Committee. But scientists realized that they were dealing with just a concept, lacking in hard data. A 1958 Committee study for the St. Louis Dairy Council on rising Stronium-90 levels in milk concluded that milk data alone was not enough to estimate the harm being done.

At virtually the same time, an article appeared in a scientific journal with a novel idea. Dr. Herman Kalckar, a biologist working for the National Institutes of Health in Washington, proposed measuring radiation in baby teeth around the world to track the extent that bomb fallout was accumulating in human bodies. Writing the August 2, 1958 issue of Nature, Kalckar laid forth the reasons behind his proposal:

> "The official public health agencies of every nation…should organize a large-scale collection of milk teeth…and conduct measurements of radioactivity on this material… Such an International Milk Teeth Radiation Census would contribute important information concerning the amount and kind of radiation received by the most sensitive section of any population, namely, the children."

Kalckar went on to note that radioactive strontium and cesium is taken up more intensely in children than in adolescents and adults. He knew well that Strontium-90 was likely to be the chemical selected for study, and that it was harmful, especially to children. Several years after his proposal, he noted in the CNI newsletter that "Strontium 90 is not an innocent contaminant; prolonged exposure can give rise to bone cancer and leukemia."

Kalckar's vision was not just to do a scientific study, but to do it with participation of large numbers of citizens:

"Such a census...would represent a simple and active type of mutual cooperation between a family unit and the scientists. At the same time, such a project would have a social touch and an aspect of cheerfulness despite the serious background of growing nuclear power."

When Kalckar's article calling for a tooth census appeared, it quickly reached the desk of Alfred Schwartz. A pediatrician at Washington University and a CNI vice-president, Schwartz was immediately struck by the idea. The government was already studying Sr-90 in bones, but it was very difficult to collect bones; they were only available on autopsy, and family permission was needed. Teeth were much easier to collect, as it meant only a donation of teeth when they were shed, typically between the ages of 6 and 13. Schwartz, thinking it a perfect project for the Committee to tackle, raised the idea with other CNI leaders.

Schwartz and his colleagues recognized that a tooth study was important to catalogue the rising levels of fallout in human bodies. They also understood that any study should start immediately. Since the Nevada testing began in 1951, children born before testing were at least eight years old and already beginning to shed baby teeth. (Scientists knew that almost all Sr-90 in a baby tooth was absorbed just before and after birth). It was critical that the study include a significant number of "pre-bomb" teeth (children born before 1951) as a baseline, so that the true buildup in fallout could be measured.

The man who Schwartz most impressed was Barry Commoner, a biology professor at Washington University and CNI founder. The CNI Executive Committee unanimously approved Commoner's proposal that CNI take on a baby tooth study at its meeting of December 10, 1958. Commoner wrote a press release, which appeared in the St. Louis Post-Dispatch eleven days later. The study, which was officially named the Baby Tooth Survey (BTS), was under way.

Although CNI scientists made up most of the BTS study leadership, their first problem was one that needed significant help from citizens - tooth collection. But before teeth could be collected, the Committee first had to decide what information was needed from each donor. While CNI scientists could have collected large amounts of data, they only selected the most important information. They wanted parents and dentists to be able to fill out forms quickly, and wanted information to fit on a 3 x 5 card. The final decision was to include the following:

Name of child
Name of parent
Address of parent
Phone number of parent
Sex of child
Date of birth
Year that tooth was lost
City and state where mother lived during last six months of pregnancy
Child's residence during the first year of life
Months on breast milk
Months on formula
Kind of milk used in formula
Other milk used in first year of life
Type of tooth (incisor, cuspid, 1st molar, 2nd molar)
Was tooth carious? (decayed)
Was tooth restored? (contained a filling)
Was the tooth's root included?

The card included the Committee's address and phone number in case parents had questions. It also included a note that "The Baby Tooth Survey is sponsored by the Greater St. Louis Committee for Nuclear Information in cooperation with the Schools of Dentistry at St. Louis and Washington University."

There were medical and statistical reasons for selecting these items:

- A child would be assigned to a certain geographic area by where they lived during pregnancy and the first year of life – not by their current address

- Trends in Sr-90 would be analyzed according to the year (even month) of birth

- Incisors, cuspids, and molars would be analyzed separately

- Teeth from breast-fed babies would be tested separately from formula-fed ones. Scientists wondered if one type of feeding brought more Sr-90 into the body

In addition, the Committee designed another 3 x 5 card to be attached to the card with information on the child. This second card gave a short summary of the Baby Tooth Study, with a description of Sr-90

> "Strontium-90 is a radioactive material in fallout from hydrogen and atomic bomb explosions. It has been increasing in food and is retained in the developing bones and teeth of children. The teeth you send will be analysed for strontium-90 so that more may be learned about the accumulation of this radioactive substance in the human body. Results will be published. Since teeth must be pooled to provide enough material for each analysis, no reports on individual teeth can be made. Please send baby teeth from children of all ages and as many teeth as possible from each child."

At the bottom of this card was a message printed in bold lettering "Send a tooth – get a button" with a picture of a boy missing teeth next to it. Sure enough, when a tooth was received, CNI staff sent each child a button with that same boy's face surrounded by the words "I gave my tooth to science."

To send the tooth, the parent was instructed to wrap the tooth in tissue or cotton and attach it to the card with tape. The two cards could be folded and sent to the Committee address, also printed on the card.

Despite a shoestring budget, committee leaders were determined not just to conduct the study, but to make it scientifically meaningful. They boldly set a goal of collecting 50,000 baby teeth in the first year, setting up the next immediate problem of making massive requests for teeth. By 1960, the Committee had printed up 1 million cards.

But even with many cards prepared, there was no guarantee that people would give teeth. Handling this issue is perhaps the greatest legacy of the St. Louis tooth study, a brilliant display of citizens assisting in a scientific project. The first efforts were modest. The St. Louis Women's Auxiliary collected and catalogued the first 3,000 teeth in January, February, and March 1959.

But the CNI went far beyond the Women's Auxiliary. Leaders appealed to the civic pride of various groups, and kept the message as non-political as possible – no dramatic outcry to stop bomb testing was made. Instead, the message was more like "let's find out how much fallout is getting into our kids bodies." Among the groups that were successfully tapped were:

St. Louis city and county public schools
St. Louis catholic schools
United Church Women
Council of Catholic Women
Council of Jewish Women
The Junior League
St. Louis Dental Society
St. Louis public libraries
St. Louis Health Department dental clinics

Schools and dentists were of critical importance. Because nearly 1.5 million people were living in St. Louis city or county, hundreds of thousands of young children were attending local schools. Typically the CNI would approach a school superintendent, asking permission to distribute 3 x 5 cards to schoolchildren to bring home to their parents, along with a pamphlet explaining the program. The first successes bred not only tooth contributions, but more successes. Dentists were also an important way to obtain teeth. Dentists would keep pamphlets and cards in their offices, and parents would pick them up and bring them home.

Yvonne Logan, who directed the BTS, described some of the innovative ways used to publicize the study and collect teeth in 1964:

> "During the weeks of the semi-annual Tooth Roundups, public service time is given generously by radio and televistion stations to publicize the needs of the Survey. Mayor Raymond Tucker has proclaimed Tooth Survey Week. Last December, the Veiled Prophet queen, St. Louis' traditional reigning beauty, celebrated the Survey's fifth birthday with a party at Children's Hospital. A large model of a tooth (with a child inside) gives out forms in department stores."

Dr. Louise Reiss, who was Logan's predecessor as study director, credits the role of volunteers to make the study successful:

> "No scientific group as such could possibly tackle the teeth collecting. It's a big, backbreaking job – this is probably the largest research study that has ever depended to such a degree on public

participation. Fortunately, we have several volunteer workers. We're going to need them all."

The CNI newsletter, entitled Scientist and Citizen, described how the Committee made use of the relatively new medium of television to reach parents:

> "The Tooth Fairy, who used to come quietly in the night, when children were asleep, now makes her appearance in full daylight – and even welcomes a blaze of publicity. She appears regularly on St. Louis TV channels in spot announcements urging children to send teeth to the Baby Tooth Survey."

The collection program was a great success. By the end of 1959, about 14,500 teeth had been collected, short of the original goal but a large number. By the end of 1961, this number had risen to over 70,000.

Years later, many parents and children recall the study.

> "I do have fond memories of having participated as a child through the donation of my baby teeth…Along with collecting the glowing tails of fireflies, sending my baby teeth off to science is something I've never forgotten about my childhood. Perhaps due to this early experience, I have been working in the field of medical research for the past 15 years."

> "I was born in St. Louis in 1954 and I have a vivid, albeit incomplete memory of being on the local news with the mayor of St. Louis regarding a promotional project that had something to do with baby teeth! I was quite young, I would guess 4 years old, not yet school age, yet old enough to have some long lasting memory of the event. If my estimate is correct, that may have been 1958 or 1959."

> "I was a member of 'Operation Tooth Club' – I gave my teeth to science. I had a card that was lost in 1980 when my wallet was stolen, and I have been sad about that to this day."

> "Sometime in the early 60s my son gave his 'tooth to science.' The reason I remember it so clearly is that the pin went through the washing machine and he was heartbroken. I contacted wherever it

was that a person contacted at that time, and he was sent another pin with a note that said 'Anything to mend a broken heart.'"

"I remember writing a note to the tooth fairy each time that the reason there were no teeth is because we donated it to science."

"My mother, Sue Leonard, drew the picture of the little boy on the button…Some of the original artwork is at one of the museums at the Smithsonian. I remember giving my tooth. I also remember the giant tooth. We had it at our house. What memories!"

"I recall the slogan "give your tooth to science" and as an elementary school child was awarded a prize for my contribution to a poster contest advertising the study!"

"Everyone I knew at my school also had their teeth donated to the St. Louis Baby Tooth Survey…at my last class reunion, many of us talked about this very same thing."

"I was featured in a 1967 or 1968 Baby Tooth Survey news item. A girl I did not know and I got to meet Mayor Alphonso Cervantes at this office in the St. Louis City Hall. We were on the evening news, with the Mayor pinning 'I Gave My Tooth to Science' buttons on our shirts and sweaters. I still have a photograph his office sent me of the event."

"My sister and I laughed at the memories of being furious at our Mom for denying the tooth fairy his (or her) due by giving away our baby teeth to some dumb doctors. Glad it made a difference."

"I am the 50,000 tooth girl. I remember going on a television show called Captain Eleven and having my picture in the paper as well as a newspaper article written about me and the project. It was real exciting at the time. My mother still has the big blue ribbon that I received."

Much of the work to make sure information was complete and accurate was done by volunteers. But only dentists could determine whether each tooth was an incisor or molar, and whether or not it was decayed. The Committee made sure that local dentists were involved by recruiting the deans of the two local dental schools, and directors of the state and local dental societies to be advisors to the project. The deans and society leaders recruited dentists to volunteer their time to complete information on the cards.

The next problem faced by the Committee was determining who would actually test the baby teeth for Sr-90. This was not an easy task, as no laboratory had any experience in this specific type of work. CNI leaders made early inquiries to private labs, which replied that costs would be very high – much higher than the Committee could afford. To get started, the Committee enlisted a New Jersey lab, Isotopes Inc. to test the first teeth, as the lab had secured a $3000 grant from Consumers Union to take the financial heat off CNI.

Testing proved to be no simple undertaking. Preparing the teeth was the first step, a process that took three weeks. Teeth were arranged into groups, according to type of tooth, month of birth, residence, and type of feeding (breast or formula). Thus, groups such as "incisors from formula-fed St. Louis children born January 1951" were formed. Working carefully, lab personnel eliminated any decay or fillings, and shaved off the roots of the teeth. Any tooth that was badly decayed was not tested.

Then there was the problem of how many teeth to test at a time. It would have been nice to test each individual tooth, but this was not possible – the machine used to count Sr-90 could not detect the chemical in such a small substance like a single baby tooth. Lab personnel figured out that 25-90 teeth tested together in a single group would be needed. But the system worked, and the first results began to trickle out of the lab.

While this was going on, CNI leaders persuaded the Dental School at Washington University to develop a machine to test large numbers of teeth. The lead researcher at the school was Dr. Harold Rosenthal. A biochemist who specialized in radioactivity, the New Jersey-born Rosenthal was an experienced researcher who saw the unique role played by the project. "We just wanted to present information to help stop bomb testing," he recalled years later. To develop the machine that would test teeth, he enlisted the help of the Argonne National Laboratory outside Chicago, which put together a large, steel-plated device that could detect relatively low levels of radiation.

As Rosenthal went about his work setting up the technical part of the study, Commoner spent considerable effort raising funds to support it. Early in the study, he raised $10,000 from the Leukemia Guild of Missouri and Illinois, and dues from the growing number of CNI members were put into the study, but much more was needed. He estimated that to be significant, the study would have to test teeth from about 10% of St. Louis schoolchildren age 5-13, who were losing teeth. This would cost about $250,000 over five years. This was a huge amount, and only one source could have covered it: the federal government. In 1959, Commoner and his colleagues persuaded the National Institute for Dental Research in Washington to commit $197,454 over the next five years. Other funds were needed, but this was the big one. The Baby Tooth Survey was now officially a "go."

The years 1959, 1960, and 1961 were especially exciting for the BTS. Teeth were being received by the thousands. CNI volunteers criss-crossed St. Louis to encourage donations. Media stories appeared, not just in local publications but national ones. The April 25, 1960 issue of Newsweek covered the progress of the study. But as time went on, the question on the minds of many persisted: what were the results?

As teeth results came in, CNI leaders were eager to make them public. But they wisely waited for a significant number of teeth to be received. They also decided to publish results in a scientific journal, rather than just through the lay media. Because journal articles must pass a "peer review" from experts in the field, publication in such a journal would give the study much greater credibility. With the military pushing so hard to achieve a superior number of nuclear weapons, the tooth study was sure to be attacked, so Committee members knew that a strong study had to be presented to weather the storm.

Committee leaders waited until a large number of teeth had been tested to put together an article. Aiming high, they decided to submit results to the journal Science. This British publication was over 100 years old, and one of the most respected scientific publications in the world. Dr. Louise Reiss emerged as the scientist that would write the article.

Reiss was an internist practicing in St. Louis. She and her husband Eric, also a physician, had become very interested in the bomb fallout issue and both had become very active in the CNI. Louise directed the Baby Tooth Study in its first three years – on a volunteer basis - and Eric had testified before Congress in 1959 of the dangers of mounting fallout. She recalled years later

> "My role in the tooth survey was specific. I was asked to set it up because I had an MD degree and my boards in internal medicine. This was expected to give me entrée to the Health Department and the two Dental Schools where approval was needed to sanctify the project as a scientific endeavor at a time of much political turmoil and paranoia.
>
> I planned the forms needed for data collection... I gave talks all over town to church groups and PTAs – and then there was TV."

She prepared a draft and submitted it to Science, and then went through the long agonizing process of waiting for an answer. Much to the delight of CNI and many in St. Louis, the answer was positive. On November 24, 1961, nearly three years to the day since the baby tooth study had begun, Science published the article. It was based on results of 1335 baby teeth that had been tested by Isotopes Inc. (Louise) Reiss had dotted all her i's and crossed all her t's. She made sure that only certain teeth were included. Only incisors from children born 1951-1954, whose mother had lived in St. Louis during pregnancy and the first year of life, were studied.

Reiss noted that children who had been breast fed for at least one month had less Sr-90 in their teeth than children who had been only fed with formula. She also noted a companion study on teeth and bones from 43 skeletons from stillborn children, and found that Sr-90 accumulates uniformly in teeth and bones – thus suggesting that baby teeth was a good marker for Sr-90 throughout the body, not just the teeth.

But the big news was the sharp rise in Sr-90 in baby teeth over time. Beginning in 1951 (the year that Nevada bomb tests began), average Sr-90 levels rose each year, until by 1954, average levels were nearly four times higher than they were in 1951. Because so many teeth had been tested, results were highly significant. In the article, Reiss downplayed the result, noting dryly that "The upward trend with time may be correlated with increasing dietary concentrations of Sr-90." She also made no mention that Sr-90 and other types of fallout might pose a cancer risk for American children.

Average Sr-90 in baby teeth, St. Louis incisors, formula fed babies
In picocuries of Sr-90 per gram of calcium

Year born	Avg. Sr-90
Last half 1951	0.188
Last half 1952	0.196
Last half 1953	0.350
Last half 1954	0.588

But the cat was now out of the bag. CNI now had hard evidence that bomb test fallout was building up in the bodies of Americans. Just over a year after the Reiss article appeared, Rosenthal published another article in Science with updated tooth figures, showing that in 1958, average Sr-90 in baby teeth was SEVEN times higher than it was in 1951. Naturally, many began to wonder about what figures would be for those born in the early 1960s.

Although the Committee was enjoying greater success, it didn't come without opposition. In a politically-charged area like atomic bomb tests, there were plenty of detractors. Their opinions were strong – any criticism of America's bomb test program would hurt national security, and impair the nation's readiness for an atomic war with the Soviet Union. Some went even farther, charging those who opposed bomb testing with having Communist sympathies. The nation had just gone through a period of hysteria in the 1950s that Communists had infiltrated much of American society. Senator Joseph McCarthy was initially successful in making this charge, until they proved to be largely exaggerated.

The paranoia that Communists were infiltrating groups opposed to bomb testing made it to a U.S. Senate subcommittee, which prepared a report in October 1960. The document identified CNI as an organization favored by Communists, along with various unions, religious groups, and advocacy groups. The CNI had always made efforts to make itself a provider of information, rather than an interest group, even though it was in close contact with groups openly opposed to bomb testing. However, the finger had been pointed, and CNI leaders rose to its defense.

The accusations became sharper the following spring, when the Senate subcommittee turned its attention to Linus Pauling, who refused to identify who helped him circulate his petition to halt bomb testing. Pauling's book No More War! identified four members of the Washington University faculty

(Martin Kamen, Leslie Dunn, Philip Morrison, and Oswald Veblen), and thus the subcommittee charged these men with

> "an unwillingness or inability, in the course of their activities, to draw the line between communists and non-communists, and/or they have, like Dr. Pauling, been consistent participants in communists-front organizations."

Right-wing groups picketed the Washington University campus that spring, dividing a community that largely supported CNI activities. The charges were never proven, and CNI continued its work, but it did cast a pall over the group's activities.

The Baby Tooth Survey had plenty of momentum to weather the charges of communism. In April 1960, the St. Louis mayor declared a "Tooth Survey Week" in the city. Several years later, a local reporter made a short film on the project. Community organizer Yvonne Logan had replaced Louise Reiss as director of the BTS, and used her experience to collect more teeth.

A big worry in the early 1960s was how to continue support of the study after the large federal grant expired. Commoner was successful in getting a $52,496 extension, which would go a long way to testing teeth into the late 1960s. Another grant, for $50,000, was obtained from the Danforth Foundation in St. Louis. Membership was soaring, to 900 by mid-1960, and a larger amount of dues were used in the project. Despite these successes, the BTS was still largely reliant on the work of hundreds of volunteers.

With the total of teeth soaring, results being published in scientific journals, and adequate funding secured for a long-term effort, the BTS enjoyed a period of great accomplishment in the early 1960s. But this was no time for rejoicing, as events around the world made the study, and all activities related to atomic bomb testing, of greatest importance.

CHAPTER 5
TOOTH STUDY SHAPES POLICY IN DEPTHS OF COLD WAR

When the United States and Soviet Union agreed to stop testing nuclear weapons in the fall of 1958, many Americans breathed a sigh of relief. The relentless parade of bombs, the worry about nuclear war, and the buildup of fallout had taken its toll. The year 1958 was especially trying; a total of 79 U.S. bombs were exploded, the most ever in a single year. A few were tested below the Nevada desert, but almost all of them were in the atmosphere.

While the truce was an uneasy one – many still saw Soviet Communism as a menace and saw nuclear war as likely – there were some bright spots. Negotiators for the two superpowers began to discuss a permanent test ban. And perhaps more importantly, stopping bomb tests reduced radiation levels. Chemicals that decayed rapidly like Iodine-131, Strontium-89, and Barium-140 disappeared completely from milk.

The longer-lasting chemicals increased as the fallout from all the 1958 tests rained down into the environment, but fell as the test moratorium continued. In St. Louis, average Sr-90 in milk fell by one third from late 1959 to late 1961. Average Cesium-137 in milk fell by two thirds. Later on, results from the Baby Tooth Survey backed up these measurements.

Average Sr-90 in St. Louis raw milk, last six months of the year
In picocuries of Sr-90 per liter of raw milk, from monthly measurements

Year	Value
1957	8.73
1958	16.02
1959	20.52
1960	15.05
1961	13.60

The other nuclear-related development that made Americans feel a bit better was the advent of the "peaceful atom." While the first use of nuclear power was military, there were other uses of radioactive chemicals. Certain chemicals can be used in medicine to diagnose and treat disease; by the early 1960s, these were being used with greater frequency by doctors. Another peaceful use was the production of electricity. With the encouragement of the federal government, 11 nuclear power reactors were operating in the U.S. by the summer of 1963, including four close to Chicago, Detroit, New

York, and Pittsburgh, with plans to build dozens more in the making.

The bomb test moratorium, while welcome to many, was an uneasy – and as it turned out, a short truce. The U.S. had been sending a series of high-flying spy planes over the Soviet Union. As part of the thawed relations, the Eisenhower Administration assured the Soviets that they had stopped these missions. But the military wanted just a little more information before they ceased, and continued to send spy planes, known as the U-2. In one of the last planned flights, Air Force pilot Frances Gary Powers left Pakistan on May 1, 1960, on his way to Norway. At an altitude of 68,000 feet over the Soviet Union, Powers' plane began to plummet (whether the plane failed or was shot down is still not certain). He bailed out and was taken prisoner by the Soviets; and while Powers was eventually returned to the U.S. in a prisoner exchange, Soviet leaders were furious with the United States.

More trouble was brewing. As Powers languished in a Soviet jail, the new Cuban leader Fidel Castro was causing great concern in Washington. A Communist, Castro had pledged his allegiance to the Soviet Union, making Cuba the only pro-Soviet country in the western hemisphere. Eisenhower's advisors were worried that the Soviets could establish themselves in Cuba, just 90 miles from Florida. This might mean helping Communist revolutions in other western nations, and worse yet, might mean Soviet nuclear weapons right in America's back yard.

Eisenhower's Central Intelligence Agency began to plan an invasion of Cuba to remove Castro. When John F. Kennedy became president in January 1961, he was informed of the plot, but did nothing to stop it. The invasion took place in the spring, but was a total failure. Not only did Castro retain power, but the Soviet leaders took the move as another hostile action by the U.S. The "grace period" in the Cold War was just about over. A summit conference between Kennedy and Soviet leader Nikita Khrushchev in Vienna did nothing to help matters. When the Soviets resumed testing on September 1, 1961, Kennedy had no choice but to resume tests as well.

The Soviet tests startled many, not just because they ended the three-year moratorium but because of their enormous power. One Soviet blast, set off at a remote site in Siberia, had the equivalent of 50 million tons of TNT. By comparison, the Hiroshima bomb had the power of only 15,000 tons, making the Soviet weapon more than 3,000 times more powerful. Fallout from this and other Soviet tests circled around the globe.

The Americans responded with by furiously testing their own bombs, at both the Nevada and south Pacific sites. In 1962, a record total of 98 bombs were exploded. Almost all tests in Nevada were underground, but all south Pacific tests were in the atmosphere. As this testing frenzy continued, radioactivity in the environment went back up again. The fast-decaying chemicals returned into the water and food. And the slow-decaying ones hit record levels, tripling from late 1961 to late 1962.

Almost immediately after testing resumed, citizens took action. A Washington DC children's book illustrator, Dagmar Wilson, was troubled by the resumption of bomb testing. Wilson, a mother of three, called some of her friends, and founded the Women Strike for Peace on September 21, 1961. The group quickly planned a one-day strike against bomb testing, and spread the word through PTAs, the League of Women Voters, and other women's groups.

Incredibly, the group caught on so fast that on November 1, just six weeks later, an estimated 100,000 supporters took part in marches organized by the group in 60 U.S. cities. At places like the White House and the United Nations, well-dressed women (often pushing baby carriages) carried signs, including those that said "Let the Children Grow" and "Pure Milk, Not Poison." The intent was clear: get the Strontium-90 out of my child's milk. Protests continued, and survived a Congressional inquest into charges that Women Strike for Peace was a Communist front – charges that were baseless. The efforts were peaceful ones; one of the many protests, in New York City in April 1962, was a prototype of marches that were to follow throughout the 1960s.

> "Thousands of peace workers and activists marched to the United Nations yesterday in an appeal to President Kennedy to cancel his decision to resume nuclear tests in the atmosphere…There were students, clergymen, writers, painters, actors, Quakers, a few beatniks, and many housewives. Some of whom pushed infants in carriages… A young man strummed his guitar and youngsters softly sang songs of peace with such words as 'O Lord, deep in my heart, I know that I do believe'… Many of the youths and women in the crowd carried blue and yellow flowers symbolic of peace."

Those opposed to bomb testing even put their beliefs to music. A popular song of the time was "What Have They Done to the Rain?" by folk singer and writer Malvina Reynolds, who was inspired by reports of Sr-90 in the environment:

Just a little rain, falling all around,
The grass lifts its head to the heavenly sound,
Just a little rain, just a little rain,
What have they done to the rain?

Just a little boy, standing in the rain,
The gentle rain that falls for years,
And the grass is gone, the boy disappears,
And rain keeps falling like helpless tears,
And what have they done to the rain?

Just a little breeze out of the sky,
The leaves pat their hands as the breeze goes by,
Just a little breeze with some smoke in its eye,
What have they done to the rain?

Words and Music by Malvina Reynolds, © 1962, Schroder Music Co.

Despite the marches, the testing went on and Cold War tensions mounted, reaching a peak in October 1962. U.S. spy planes had photographed Soviet missile bases being built in Cuba. Nuclear weapons launched from these sites could easily strike all major American cities. Kennedy announced a naval blockade of the waters around Cuba, and demanded that the Soviets remove the missile bases. After several days in which the world teetered on the brink of nuclear war, an agreement was reached and the missile bases were removed. The world breathed a sigh of relief after the near-holocaust.

Kennedy had been a supporter of a ban on nuclear tests even before he became president. The resumption of tests and the Cuban Missile Crisis had disturbed him greatly. Kennedy's science advisor Jerome Wiesner related a conversation with Kennedy on radioactive fallout as the president looked out the window on a rainy day.

> "And I told him that it was washed out of the clouds by the rain, that it would be brought to earth by rain, and he said, looking out the window, 'You mean it's in the rain out there?' – and I said 'Yes'; and he looked out the window, looked very sad, and didn't say a word for several minutes."

After the Cuban crisis, Kennedy instructed his negotiating team of the critical need for a test ban. Within months, an agreement was reached between the U.S., Soviet Union, and Great Britain, that called for an end to all nuclear tests above the ground and in the water. In an appeal to the U.S. Senate to ratify the treaty, Kennedy spoke to the nation about the grim realities of bomb fallout on children's health:

> "This treaty can be a step towards freeing the world from the fears and dangers of radioactive fallout… Continued unrestricted testing, by the nuclear powers, joined in time by other nations which may be less adept in limiting pollution, will increasingly contaminate the air that all of us must breathe.
>
> Even then, the number of children and grandchildren with cancer in their bones, with leukemia in their blood, or with poison in their lungs might seem statistically small to some, in comparison with natural health hazards. But this is not a natural health hazard, and it is not a statistical issue. The loss of even one human life, or the malformation of even one baby, who may be born long after we are gone, should be of concern to us all. Our children and grandchildren are not merely statistics toward which we can be indifferent."

The Senate easily endorsed the treaty by an 80-19 vote, and Kennedy signed it, just one month before he was assassinated. While China and France continued to test nuclear weapons above the ground until 1980, there were many fewer such tests. The era of large-scale weapons testing was over, and the world breathed a sigh of relief. Lyndon Johnson, who had succeeded Kennedy as president, outlined just how the treaty had greatly reduced what was perhaps the greatest threat to the world:

> "We cannot and we will not abandon the test ban treaty…since this agreement was signed and the tests stopped, the dread strontium-89 and iodine-131 have disappeared from the environment. The amount of strontium-90 and cesium-137 has already been, in 1 year, cut in half. This is technical language, but what it means is that we can breathe safely again."

But the damage had been done. Radioactivity from the flurry of bomb testing in the early 1960s reached the stratosphere and rained into the environment. The slow-decaying chemicals took several years to completely return to earth, and levels in the food chain climbed steadily, reaching a peak in the spring of 1964. In this period, average levels of Sr-90 in milk were more than three times higher than the spring of 1961. Levels of Cesium-137 were nearly ten times higher. With no new tests, levels began to fall after that, but only gradually.

The general belief that during the 1950s and early 1960s were prosperous, and that the health of Baby Boomers was the best of any group of American children in history does not stand up to the facts. Although public health experts were silent, the following happened in these years – the years of above-ground atomic bomb testing.

- Infant deaths, which had been dropping rapidly for years, only fell 13% in the U.S. from 1950 to 1965, the poorest record of the entire 20th century. In the years 1952, 1957, 1958, and 1962 – all years of large-scale bomb tests the rate actually increased from the prior year.

- The national rate of low-weight births, rose 2% for whites and 35% for non-whites from 1950 to 1966. A baby born under normal weight, or 5½ pounds, is often the result of a premature delivery.

- The rate of fetal deaths, or stillbirths, declined only 14% from 1950-1964, even though it declined much more rapidly during all years before and after during the 20th century.

- Although no registry of birth defects was kept during these years, the U.S. death rate from such defects for children age 5-14 rose 53% from 1950 to 1960.

This poor record of infant and child health extended to cancer. In the early 1960s childhood cancer rates reached an all-time high. Nationwide, the 1962-63 cancer death rate for children age 19 and under was 8.0 per 100,000 persons, up 40% from the 5.7 rate of 1937-38. The incidence rate for the same periods in Connecticut, the only state with a reliable cancer registry, was up a staggering 90% (8.0 to 15.3 per 100,000). While a generation ago, about 2,600 children died each year from cancer, the figure had now reached 5,700.

Each and every case of cancer in children was an agony, mostly for the child but also for friends and family. Leukemia was the most common type of cancer among children, accounting for nearly half of the deaths. Leukemia is a disease of the white blood cells in bone marrow tissue. Although it had first been identified by doctors in 1845, it was a virtual death sentence over a century later, as most children only lived for several months after diagnosis. There was no way to detect the disease early, nor to treat it. A child would typically show a number of symptoms that didn't seem to be connected: fevers, frequent infections, anemia, shortness of breath, unusual bruising or bleeding, bone and joint pain, swollen glands, and poor appetite. George W. Bush's sister Robin was one such victim. The little three-year old girl was diagnosed in February 1952; despite the best care available at that time, she died just eight months later.

The child cancer situation was getting so bad, that medical leaders scrambled quickly to do something about it. Dr. Sidney Farber, a pathologist at Children's Hospital in Boston, founded a free clinic for children with cancer. The Variety Club in Boston heard about Farber's efforts and established the Children's Cancer Research Foundation to fund the clinic. Farber and the Foundation jump started their cause on May 22, 1948, on the radio program "Truth or Consequences" when it switched to a Boston hospital to introduce Carl Einar Gustafson, a young boy with cancer. Farber, seeking to protect the child's identity, gave the boy the name Jimmy for the show, and unwittingly gave the name to the soon-to-be-famous Jimmy Fund. Program host Ralph Edwards sent out a pitch to America, not just for Jimmy, but for all children with cancer:

> "Folks, Jimmy doesn't know he has cancer. And we're not using any photographs of him or giving his full name so he will know about it."

The show was a terrific success, as many Americans sent telegrams and donated money to the cause. Members of the Boston Braves baseball team visited Gustafson, and Red Sox star Ted Williams soon dedicated himself to the cause. Gustafson, who had cancer in his stomach, recovered to live a full life, hold down a job as a truck driver, and have a family.

Others joined the bandwagon to stop the childhood cancer menace. Danny Thomas, the television star who prayed to St. Jude Thaddeus, the patron saint of hopeless causes, became very involved with the disease. In 1957, Thomas (who was of Lebanese descent) formed the American Lebanese Syrian

Associated Charities to help raise money for research and treatment.

Five years later, Thomas helped open the St. Jude Children's Research Hospital in Memphis, which is still one of the most eminent child cancer centers in the U.S.

Some physicians pioneered research into chemotherapy for youngsters, piggybacking on to the rising medical research effort sponsored by drug companies and the federal government. Thanks to efforts by Farber and others, the first new drugs for treating children with leukemia were introduced in the mid-1950s. They extended a stricken child's life expectancy from just 3 to 6 months, but it was a start.

The massive effort to treat children with cancer was not matched by an effort to understand what caused the disease. Of the several theories that began to circulate in the medical and public health world, the most common one was radiation exposure. Several research studies were published that made it clearer than ever that radiation caused cancer in humans, especially in children.

The first study, of pelvic X-rays to pregnant women, was done by Alice Stewart in 1956. Stewart, a British physician assigned the task to determine what was causing a rise in childhood leukemia, conducted a survey and found that women who received a pelvic X-ray during pregnancy had nearly twice the risk of having a child who would die of cancer by age ten. The findings were very clear, although surprising, to Stewart:

> "We could see it quite early on, from the first thirty-five pairs: *yes* was turning up three times for every dead child to once for every live child, for the question 'had you had an obstetric x-ray?' And the dose was very small, very brief, a single diagnostic x-ray, a tiny fraction of the radiation exposure considered safe, and it wasn't repeated. It was enough to almost double the risk of an early cancer death…None of us had the slightest clue that this tiny dose of x-ray occurring before birth might have this powerful effect initiating childhood cancer."

Stewart published her results in the esteemed medical journal Lancet, but the reaction from many professionals was strongly negative, as she recalled years later:

"A reaction set in and the mood changed. It was as though I'd trodden on somebody's corns. The medical profession didn't like it. The obstetricians came down on me like a ton of bricks – how dare I say that x-rays are dangerous? They saw me as interfering with their practices. The radiologists were oddly divided…but most thought I was taking the bread out of their mouths – they were afraid people would stop using x-rays."

The furor over Stewart's research persisted even as she published a more detailed article in 1958. But in 1962, those who didn't believe that X-rays to pregnant women were harmful received a big setback. In that year, Harvard public health professor Brian MacMahon published an article in the Journal of the National Cancer Institute. MacMahon's research agreed with what Stewart had found, and his study was much more comprehensive. He examined records of over 700,000 children born in 37 hospitals in New York and New England from 1947-1954.

In 1963, another publication further upheld Stewart. Westinghouse physicist Ernest Sternglass wrote an article in the journal Science in which he reviewed the work of both Stewart and MacMahon. Sternglass concluded that about 5 to 10% of all childhood cancers were due to natural radiation – not that from nuclear weapons and reactors, but that found in the air, rocks, and soil.

In 1966, the National Cancer Institute published research on effects of pre-birth X-rays. The Institute had conducted a large study in New York state, Baltimore, and Minneapolis-St. Paul. Its scientists found that not only did X-rays to pregnant women cause an increase in cancer risk to children, but X-rays before conception to either the father or mother also raised risk. The process to end pelvic X-rays to expecting mothers now had momentum. Even though doctors continued to give X-rays to about 8% of pregnant women, nobody could say that the warnings about cancer risk were just a matter of Stewart's bias.

Research on health risks to children of X-rays was far ahead of research on nuclear weapon fallout. Research tracking Japanese people who survived the blasts at Hiroshima and Nagasaki started slowly; but more information was becoming available. It had been nearly 20 years since the bombs were dropped, and a growing number of medical journal articles showed that survivors had a higher rate of cancer and other diseases than did the general population of Japan.

Research on risks to people who were exposed to fallout from atomic bomb tests was virtually nil by the early 1960s. Although many tests had been conducted by the Soviet Union - a total of 219 in all, slightly more than the 206 by the U.S. – the repressive Soviet government stifled all attempts to understand health threats. In the United States, a much freer society than the Soviet Union, the situation was not much different. Government officials, still fighting a Cold War replete with nuclear weapons, were not about to admit that their program was harming its people. This party line was total. Even those who warned about fallout and supported the Test Ban Treaty would not step over the line and acknowledge that bomb tests had harmed Americans. At a 1963 press conference, just before the Test Ban Treaty was ratified by the Senate, President Kennedy sidestepped a question about fallout's hazards:

> "Mr. President, in this connection, Utah scientists have announced that Utah children under 2 years have received from 2 to 28 times as much radioactive iodine-131 last year in less than a month as our Government says is safe for an entire year. Does the Government have any plans to examine some of these children to detect possible danger?"

> "Well, I have seen the report about the radioiodine, and it is a matter of concern. As you know, the report is not unanimous. There is some controversy about it. In addition, the standards that were set do not – I don't think we should mislead the people there, that there is evidence on hand of a serious deterioration there. But, of course, it is a matter of concern to us that we not continue. But we are looking into it. But I would say that as of now that we do not believe that the health of the children involved has been adversely affected. But it does tell us – though of course these matters require further study – what it does tell us it is very desirable to get a test ban."

The government agency that was charged with stopping any information suggesting bomb test fallout caused cancer in humans was the Atomic Energy Commission. During the early 1960s, the AEC suppressed internal reports from several of its scientists that concluded those who lived downwind in Utah had been harmed. (This information was only released to the public in 1979 from requests under the Freedom of Information Act, a post-Watergate law used to make government more accountable).

One of the AEC scientists who saw his work squelched was Dr. Harold Knapp. A veterinarian, Dr. Knapp recounted his conversation with the AEC Director of Occupational Safety:

> "When I told him how high the dosage levels were, the director had this pitch: 'Well, look, we've told these people all along that it's safe and we can't change our story now; we'll be in trouble.'"

Another AEC scientist that examined bomb fallout damage was Edward Weiss. In 1965, Weiss prepared an internal report for the AEC on leukemia deaths in southwest Utah. Weiss uncovered a cluster of six leukemia deaths in Washington and Iron Counties, many times above the U.S. rate. The AEC hid the Weiss report.

The AEC cover-up extended to all branches of government. The National Institutes of Health, which gives millions in medical research grants each year, chose not to fund, nor to encourage, research on bomb fallout health effects. University-based medical centers, which were heavily dependent on government grants, chose not to rock the boat and also did not pursue studies on the subject. Without adequate financing, studies could not be conducted, and medical journals had nothing to publish. The ice was finally broken in October 1967, when Weiss published an article in the American Journal of Public Health. He found that in 1958-1962, there were 14 thyroid cancer cases diagnosed in Utah children, three times the national rate. One decade prior, before Nevada bomb testing began, only one childhood thyroid cancer case was diagnosed in the state. Thyroid cancer is strongly affected by radioactive iodine, one of the harmful chemicals in the bomb fallout clouds.

But while the government obstructed, and while the scientific community dragged its feet, people continued to press for answers in light of the growing menace of childhood cancer. Anecdotes from Utah residents who had been closest to and directly in the path of the fallout clouds mounted. The concerns also were part of the St. Louis Baby Tooth Survey. A 1960 article in Newsweek magazine on the study posed the question that many were asking as teeth were collected and tested:

> "But what about the children who have done their growing while strontium-90 levels were high – are they liable to develop cancer? No one can answer with certainty, but St. Louis's 'Operation Tooth' is one way scientists have of finding out."

CHAPTER 6
ST. LOUIS TOOTH STUDY – LATER YEARS

The early and mid-1960s was an exciting time for the Baby Tooth Survey. The number of teeth received by the Committee at their small office on Delmar Street in St. Louis soared, and reached an incredible 150,000 by June 1964. Volunteers buzzed around the city asking for help in collecting teeth. Scientists gave many talks to community groups on the risks of bomb fallout and the importance of the BTS. The political developments such as the American-Soviet struggle over Cuba, the resumption of bomb testing, and the call for a ban on testing only fueled the desire to continue the study.

The lab at Washington University was going full throttle to test baby teeth for Strontium-90. Lab director Harold Rosenthal had the crucial job of setting up testing procedures that would result in accurate and meaningful results. He made a difficult but correct decision at the outset: the Strontium-90 level in each tooth could not be calculated, and thus parents would not know the radiation burden of their child. Instead, groups of teeth were tested at one time, since the greater amount of enamel would produce an accurate result.

"We used batches of 20 incisors each, and 4 molars each, with 15 batches for each birth year" Rosenthal recalled years later. "We used a representative sample for each type of tooth for each year," he explained. Teeth were separated by type of tooth, birth month, whether a tooth had decay, residence during pregnancy and first year of life, and presence or absence of breast feeding. One batch might be 20 incisor teeth (none with decay) of children born in St. Louis in January 1957 who were never breast fed.

"The machine could test 5 or 6 batches at a time," Rosenthal said. "Each sample took a long time, about a month," he remembered. After teeth were tested, Rosenthal and his colleagues examined the results to ensure that the process and results made sense.

Two scientific calculations were needed to produce results. First, the machine had to count the level of Sr-90. This was not a matter of weight, as radioactivity is measured by the decay level. The Washington University machine, which operated like a special type of Geiger counter, produced this result. The measurement was in picocuries – one picocurie is one-trillionth of a curie.

In addition, the lab needed to measure the amount of calcium in each batch of teeth, which was a more basic process of weighing the teeth. The calcium result was measured in grams. The two numbers were used to produce a ratio of strontium-to-calcium.

Louise Reiss had written the first medical journal article on tooth study results. After she left CNI in 1962, Rosenthal took on this task. Knowing how important it was for the scientific credibility of the study, he published over a dozen pieces throughout the rest of the 1960s. And he wasted no time, knowing that results could have an effect on the debate over the Test Ban Treaty.

In the spring of 1963, he published an article in the journal Science, with the latest results of the study. He showed that in decay-free incisors St. Louis children never breast fed who were born in 1951, at the start of bomb testing, there was an average of 0.30 picocuries of Sr-90 per gram of calcium. This number had risen steadily, reaching a mark of 2.56 for children born in 1957 ---- over eight times greater than 1951 births!!! The fact that the recent resumption in bomb testing had raised radioactivity levels in milk meant that children born in the early 1960s were going to have an even greater level – an unpleasant truth that nonetheless was what CNI leaders wanted to tell the public.

In August 1964, Rosenthal followed with another article in the journal Nature. He had some good news to report, specifically that children who were breast fed at least six months had average Sr-90 levels nearly 40% below those who were breast fed less than 1½ weeks (or not at all). The belief of many scientists that breast milk would let less Sr-90 into the child's body than formula was upheld.

But Rosenthal also had some bad news to report in the article, news that was nonetheless expected. The Washington University team had to wait until a child was at least six years old for baby teeth to be shed, so results of teeth of children born during the dark days of large-scale bomb testing in 1961-62 wouldn't be available until nearly 1970. So the team set up a program of testing jaw bones and tooth buds of fetuses that had been stillborn, which would immediately produce information on the radiation burden. Sure enough, average Sr-90 levels in fetal bone and teeth had doubled from 1961 to 1963, which reflected the doubling of Sr-90 levels in milk. The darkest fears of scientists and citizens were all being confirmed.

While the St. Louis Baby Tooth Survey continued, political events were occurring towards an agreement to ban any further nuclear weapons tests in the atmosphere. After negotiators for the U.S., Soviet Union, and Great Britain agreed to the treaty, the U.S. Senate still had to ratify it. In August 1963, a Senate committee heard testimony from experts. Some of them were against the treaty, including the renowned physicist Edward Teller, a Hungarian refugee from the Nazis and an ardent cold warrior. Teller scoffed at the notion that fallout was harmful to infants and children:

> "From the present levels of world-wide fallout there is no danger. The real danger is that you will frighten mothers from giving milk to their babies. By that, probably much more damage has been done than by anything else concerning this matter."

But scientists supporting the treaty were called to testify as well. Eric Reiss, the St. Louis physician and co-founder of CNI, gave a strong statement on the health risks of fallout:

> "Our analysis of the same monitoring data published by the AEC shows that as a result of nuclear tests at the Nevada Test Site, in the period 1951-62, a number of local populations, especially in Nevada, Utah, and Idaho and probably other communities scattered throughout the continental United States, have been exposed to fallout so intense as to represent a medically unacceptable hazard to children who may drink fresh locally produced milk."

Reiss continued by saying that milk and other contaminated food products were actually entering the bodies of American children and building up rapidly – and used the Baby Tooth Survey as evidence. Soon after the testimony ended, the Senate voted to endorse the Test Ban Treaty, and President Kennedy signed it. The hopes of many who had created and worked on the tooth study had been realized. It had become an important tool in what might have been the most crucial treaty of the 20th century.

While the treaty was passed partly over fear of nuclear war, concern over fallout harming humans was clearly in the forefront. Commoner gave his opinion on the matter:

> "Many people were surprised at the ease with which the 1963 test-ban treaty was approved by the United States Senate. Several observers

have noted a possible connection with the numerous letters received by Senators from housewives and mothers who not only wanted the treaty approved but could cite serious scientific grounds for their belief that it would help reduce the medical hazards from fallout."

The Test Ban Treaty actually took away the primary goal of the St. Louis Committee. Some saw no need to continue with the group, and the membership sagged to 450 by 1965. Two years after that, CNI leaders voted to change the group's name to the Committee for Environmental Information, giving it a broader spectrum of environmental issues to tackle.

Even though the treaty had been passed, the tooth study continued on throughout the 1960s. By 1967, the number of teeth collected reached the 250,000 mark. Rosenthal's lab was now proficiently churning out results. Given that the Committee had grants totaling over $100,000 from the U.S. Public Health Service and Danforth Foundation, plus other grants and a still-eager group of volunteers, the work continued.

The St. Louis tooth study became so well known that programs in other areas were started. Rosenthal's lab received and tested teeth from a variety of regions, and found that St. Louis had one of the highest levels of Sr-90 in the nation. On the other hand, levels in California were just over half what they were in St. Louis, because prevailing winds from Nevada blew east, and generally away from California to the west.

Average Levels of Sr-90 (in picocuries per gram calcium)
Deciduous incisors of bottle fed children, born 1957

Area	Avg. Sr-90
East Texas and New Orleans	3.43
St. Louis	2.79
Indianapolis and Chicago	2.77
Michigan	2.47
Toronto	1.96
California	1.53

The St. Louis study sparked other tooth projects across the world. Scientists in Czechoslovakia, Denmark, England and Wales, Finland, the Faroe Islands, Greenland, Italy, and Norway all found what the St. Louis committee had discovered – that Sr-90 in baby teeth rose rapidly as testing went on. The study in Finland was one of the larger ones, with 5,400 baby teeth collected from 1960 to 1970. The Institute of Dentistry at the University of Helsinki, with support from the Finnish Dental Society, and religious groups, teachers, and dentists all collected teeth. Not only did it document a sharp rise in average Sr-90 over time, it also showed a lower level in incisors compared to molars, similar to what Rosenthal's lab found.

At the 1969 Radiobiological Symposium held at the Hanford nuclear weapons plant in Richland, Washington, Rosenthal provided what were the final totals of the study. Sure enough, average Sr-90 levels in St. Louis baby teeth rose each year since 1950, with the exception of the moratorium period. The peak came for St. Louis children born in 1964; the average concentration was 9.0 and 14.6 picocuries of Sr-90 per gram of calcium for incisors and molars, respectively. For children born 1951, both figures were below 1.0. This meant that children born in 1964 had at least 20 times, maybe up to 80 times, the radiation burden in their bodies as did those born before bomb testing began.

Rosenthal's article gave more bad news by showing the rapid rise in Sr-90 in the bones of fetuses during bomb testing. But it also gave some good news: after the Test Ban Treaty went into effect, smaller and smaller amounts of Sr-90 were detected in bones each year. Stillbirths in late 1968 had less than half of the Sr-90 than did those born four years earlier. No more tests meant less radiation damaging the bodies and health of children.

Now that above-ground testing had ended, those who had begun to measure radioactivity in the environment and the body all began to show fast-dropping levels. Those fast-decaying chemicals (such as Iodine-131, with a half life of 8 days) virtually disappeared. Those with longer half lives such as Sr-90 (28.7 years) were still present but in rapidly dropping quantities. In general, levels fell by about 50% from the 1963-1964 peak to the end of the 1960s.

1. Average Sr-90 in mandible bones in St. Louis stillborn fetuses dropped from 6.0 to 2.7 (picocuries Sr-90 per gram calcium) from late 1964 to late 1968

2. Average Sr-90 in bones of U.S. children age 0-4 fell from 4.25 to 2.01 (picocuries Sr-90 per gram calcium) from 1964-1971.

3. Average Sr-90 in bones of New York City adults fell from 2.2 to 1.0 (picocuries Sr-90 per gram calcium) from 1965-1974 (and 1.2 to 0.6 in San Francisco).

4. Average Sr-90 in milk in nine U.S. cities, which roughly approximates the national average, fell from 24 to 6 (picocuries Sr-90 per liter milk) from 1964-1970

As levels of radioactivity fell across the U.S. in the mid and late 1960s, there was a curiously similar reduction in rates of disease and death for American children. After 1964, the infant mortality rate began to fall sharply each year, just as it had before 1950. The rate of babies born less than 5 ½ pounds plunged as well, as did the rate of stillbirths.

Cancer rates in children also plunged, both incidence (newly diagnosed cases) and mortality (deaths). Connecticut was still the only state with a reliable registry that reported cancer cases, and a sharp plunge occurred after the testing stopped. The greatest decline took place in the youngest children, diagnosed before their 5th birthday. The record total of 60 cases in 1962 was cut in half (to 30) by 1968, and the rate returned to what it had been before bomb test fallout from Nevada began to enter the diet and body.

During Bomb Testing

Year	Cases
1962	60
1963	58
1964	53

After Bomb Testing Halt

Year	Cases
1965	38
1966	43
1967	43
1968	30

With fewer children developing cancer, and with treatment methods improving rapidly, the cancer death rate among American children plunged as well. From 1963-1970, as levels of radioactivity in the environment and body shrank, the death rate shrank as well. The rate plunged an amazing

25%, from 9.08 to 6.85 deaths per 100,000. It turns out that even though childhood cancer deaths continued to fall throughout the rest of the 20th century, the period after bomb testing was halted would be the sharpest drop ever. Below is the U.S. cancer death rate age 0-9 from 1963-2005.

Year	Deaths	Rate/100,000
1963	3489	9.08
1965	3106	8.16
1970	2542	6.85
1975	1769	5.04
1980	1463	4.43
1985	1264	3.64
1990	1172	3.22
1995	1081	2.76
2000	1001	2.52
2005	937	2.35

The ability to save children became one of the highlights of the cancer research industry. About a quarter million Americans living today have survived childhood cancer.

In January 1968, the tooth project encountered possibly its greatest threat ever. On a cold winter night, a large fire broke out in Committee offices on Delmar Street. Virtually all equipment, furniture, and books were destroyed. Amazingly, firefighters were able to throw out many boxes containing baby teeth and information cards into an alley next to the office. Volunteers and staff who were notified and raced to the scene were able to break many of these boxes free from the ice and save the treasured teeth. Some cards were burned and had to be thrown out, but amazingly over 80% of the teeth, over 100,000 in all, were saved and stored at the Committee's new office.

In 1970, funding from the Public Health Service and Danforth Foundation expired. The tooth project still had an amazingly great public profile within St. Louis, but CNI leaders believed that it was time for the study to end. All objectives had been met; a large number of teeth had been tested. The buildup of Sr-90 in bodies during above-ground bomb testing had been demonstrated. The sharp drop after testing ended was also shown. Results had been published in medical and scientific journals.

Perhaps most importantly, the tooth study had helped pass the Test Ban Treaty, which may have saved thousands of American lives. "Many of us worked on the Baby Tooth Survey, as I think did the founders, with the idea of doing our best to force the Test Ban Treaty" explained Logan. Rosenthal put it more bluntly: "We had done our job" he recollected.

In January 1971, the Committee made it official, yielding control of the study to the Washington University School of Dentistry. The remaining teeth were placed in storage. Nobody knows exactly how many teeth had been collected. "I think it was about 500,000" said Sophie Goodman, an active volunteer for the Committee. A more accurate estimate would be just over 300,000, according to numbers published in the CNI newsletter, Science and Citizen.

Naturally, the end of the St. Louis study left the country without a program measuring radioactivity levels in teeth. Measurements by the federal and state governments of levels in the environment (air, water, milk, soil, etc.) continued, but the tooth study was not picked up by the government. The end of bomb testing and the rapid drop in radioactivity across the nation had reduced, but not ended, the greatest man-made threat to human health

Government officials relaxed their mandates to monitor radioactivity. In 1971, the program measuring Sr-90 levels in bones of children ended after 10 years and 3,000 samples. In 1982, tests of adult bones from New York City and San Francisco ended after nearly 30 years. The U.S. now had no means of understanding how much radioactivity was entering the bodies of its citizens.

Many considered passage of the Test Ban Treaty to be the most important purpose of the tooth study. But there were other questions. Had Americans been harmed by the fallout? Did absorbing this radiation cause some children to develop cancer? Were there any other health problems caused by fallout? New studies on humans had to be done. Dr. H.T. Blumenthal MD PhD, writing in a 1964 issue of the CNI newsletter commented "there is a certain way of translating information from animal experiments to the human situation." This would be a long and difficult task.

The topic was certainly debated within CNI. "We wanted to do a 10-15 year followup health study," said Yvonne Logan, who directed the study in the early 1960s. "We always said the value of the research could only be borne out by tracking the same children 15 years later." Commoner wanted to test teeth individually, so that a Sr-90 level could be assigned to each child. But Rosenthal refused, because accurate Sr-90 levels could only be obtained by testing batches of teeth put together - his machine could not calculate an accurate measurement for something as tiny as a single baby tooth. So no follow up health study using the St. Louis teeth was possible.

But such a study could be done using larger sized samples. Because tests of Sr-90 in bone typically examined jaw bones or spines, they were certainly large enough. As it turned out, at least three "case control" studies were done in the 1960s. This study compared people with and without a disease. The three studies examined Sr-90 in bones of people with and without cancer. One took place in the U.S., and the others in Japan and Poland.

Even though each was published in a medical journal, not much was learned from these studies. Samples sizes were small, and included few children. The largest study, the one by Japanese scientists, included 6 children who died from leukemia before age ten. Average Sr-90 in their upper leg bones were 46% greater than those for young children who died from a cause other than leukemia. But these studies certainly were not enough to make a judgment call.

And so the bomb test era ended without any understanding about how all the fallout had harmed Americans. Even those Utah and Nevada residents living close to the test site who suffered from cancer got no recognition from federal authorities that fallout had been the cause. The issue was discarded – at least for now.

The St. Louis Baby Tooth Survey left several legacies. It made its mark in the scientific world, as it became the largest study of in-body radioactivity in the world. Scientists from many nations took note of it and simultaneously did similar studies. In future years, other studies of Sr-90 in baby teeth would copy it as well.

It made its mark in the political arena. Results were used to educate the public, not just in St. Louis but around the country, about the rapid buildup of bomb test fallout. In the end, it helped bring about a halt to nuclear weapons testing above the ground. There was a split decision over whether the study was more science or politics. "We tried to stick with science and to leave politics out of it" said Reiss, but as Rosenthal put it "What we did was very political."

It became an integral part of the St. Louis community. In 2001, over 40 years after the study began, Rosenthal stated that "I've run into a lot of people who donated teeth who remember the study from their button." He added that at a recent meeting of Washington University "Several people came up to me at the Washington University emeritus meeting in mid-November, and told me their kids had donated teeth."

But the tooth project also established a prototype for scientists working with citizens for the improvement of scientific knowledge and the betterment of the public at large. Before the atomic era, scientific knowledge was relatively unsophisticated compared to what it is today. But in several areas, including atomic energy, huge technological gains have been made – gains that affect the lives of all people. Thus, it is important that people become involved in these areas, or risk a scientific elite making decisions for them.

Louise Reiss pointed proudly to the special role that citizens can play in understanding science and translating that knowledge into policy. "I continue to be moved by knowledge that a group of organized people can effectively pressure the government if they come with data instead of rhetoric" she wrote in 1996. Commoner, writing in his book Science and Survival, may have best expressed the value of this landmark effort:

> "When it became known that scientists were willing to try to explain the fallout problem, we were besieged with questions… And every lecture led to demands for more. Many of us became heavily engaged in the community's lecture circuit: PTAs, Lions, Rotarians, forums, television interviews… We saw at first hand the great need for providing the public with the information that every citizen must have if he is to decide for himself what policies our nation and the world should follow with respect to nuclear testing, civil defense, and disarmament.
>
> The children who gave up the traditional visit of the tooth fairy to contribute their baby teeth to science were in this case helping to develop new scientific information for their own future welfare."

CHAPTER 7
REACTORS RE-KINDLE INTEREST IN RADIATION HEALTH

In 1953, new President Dwight D. Eisenhower met with his advisors. Something had to be done about the growing fear of atomic energy. The race for nuclear weapon superiority with the Soviet Union was going at full speed. People were becoming increasingly aware that an attack of nuclear weapons could kill millions of Americans. They were also more aware that each bomb test in Nevada and the Pacific spread harmful fallout through the environment and entered people's bodies through breathing and the food chain.

The nation needed to understand that atomic energy was not just for warfare, that there were other, less destructive uses. One of these uses was the ability of atomic energy to generate electricity. Scientists had discovered that the great heat created when bombarding uranium atoms with neutrons could be transformed into electricity through turbines. Because most electricity to that time was produced by burning coal, a dirty and polluting process, nuclear power offered another, potentially cleaner option.

On December 8, 1953, Eisenhower addressed the United Nations with an eloquent plea for the United States to distribute nuclear material around the world to

> "serve the peaceful pursuits of mankind. Experts would be mobilized to apply atomic energy to the needs of agriculture, medicine, and other peaceful activities. A special purpose would be to provide abundant electrical energy in the power-starved areas of the world. Thus the contributing powers would be dedicating some of their strength to serve the needs rather than the fears of mankind."

The term "peaceful atom" now was in circulation. Eisenhower quickly moved to ask Congress for its help. The 1954 Atomic Energy Act allowed utility companies to develop these reactors. Uranium, the same uranium used in atomic bombs, would fuel the reactors. The federal Atomic Energy Commission was given regulatory authority over all nuclear power reactors.

The AEC became the government mouthpiece for private development of atomic power. Reactors were a favorite of the AEC. In a 1954 speech, AEC

Chairman Lewis Strauss used the term "too cheap to meter" that would characterize – and later haunt – the nuclear power industry:

> "It is not too much to expect that our children will enjoy electrical energy too cheap to meter – will know of great periodic regional famines only as matters of history- will travel effortlessly over the seas and under them and through the air with a minimum of danger and at great speeds – and will experience a lifespan far longer than ours, as disease yields and man comes to understand what causes him to age. This is the forecast for an age of peace."

Government cheerleading to promote the "peaceful atom" included directly reaching out to some of its powerful supporters. One of these was TV, movie, and amusement park chief Walt Disney, who had long been involved in public affairs. Government officials met with Disney about using his media apparatus to inform Americans about how atomic power really helped the world's people, rather than pose a threat to its existence. A December 1955 meeting with Disney brought a favorable response, and an animated cartoon on atomic power began.

Disney advisor Dr. Heinz Haber was an astrophysicist who had served in the Nazi air force, the Luftwaffe, during World War II. Haber collaborated with the U.S. Navy and General Dynamics (which built nuclear-powered submarines) and delivered a 60-minute animated cartoon based on a new book entitled "Our Friend the Atom." The story began with a fisherman who opens a bottle. A genie emerges, and tells the fisherman that he will kill anyone who released him. After tricking the genie back into its bottle, the fisherman convinces the genie to grant his wishes if he frees him again. The parallel to atomic energy is obvious. The rest of the film describes the potential uses of the atom, including the prediction that "clean" nuclear reactors would someday replace the "dirty" oil and coal plants. Reactors, and other uses such as medicine, agriculture, and household items, represent "our chance to make the atomic genie our friend." The film was released in January 1957 to a curious American public.

Despite the public relations push, the expected surge of private companies who wanted to build nuclear reactors didn't happen. Electrical utilities knew that reactors used uranium, and produced the same mix of 100-plus radioactive chemicals found in nuclear weapon explosions. They had to maintain this radioactivity within the reactor, and keep it from being released. A 1957 study by the Brookhaven National Laboratories confirmed that thousands would die or become sick after such a release. Not only would the damage be terrible, law suits seeking damages would probably bankrupt the company.

Once again, it was government to the rescue. Congress quickly passed the Price-Anderson Act in 1957. The law limited liability payments from a utility in case of a major accident to $600 million – even though actual costs might be much greater. Anything beyond $600 million would be picked up by the taxpayers.

With this bailout, utilities began ordering reactors. The first one built was Shippingport, just outside of Pittsburgh. From Denver, President Eisenhower waved a magic wand to activate an automated shovel to officially begin construction. The design for Shippingport was given to the Westinghouse company by the Navy, which used the same design for its nuclear-powered submarines. The reactor was small, and took just two years to construct. In December 1957, the reactor had been fully tested and became the first commercial nuclear power reactor in the world to produce electricity.

In the years to follow, other reactors began operating. Among the earliest ones were reactors located close to major cities, including (along with Pittsburgh) Chicago, New York, and Detroit. Actually, only a small portion of planned reactors in those early days ever operated. Some utilities were rather rambunctious in their proposals. New York City, the largest city in the nation with just under 8 million people, was targeted for many reactors by the Consolidated Edison company, including

- a reactor under Central Park in the middle of Manhattan
- a reactor under Roosevelt Island, in the East River just off Manhattan
- a reactor in Queens, just across the East River from Manhattan
- eight reactors on two manmade islands off Coney Island, the southern part of the city

Con Edison officially applied to the AEC to build the reactor in Queens, called Ravenswood, in 1962. Reaction was strong, even from those who supported nuclear power. Citizens organized and held public hearings, complete with sayings like "Why gamble with the safety of 10 million people?" When Con Edison finally withdrew its proposal in 1964, former AEC chairman David Lilienthal applauded the decision, saying it "affects the whole future of nuclear power in urban centers throughout the U.S." Sure enough, no nuclear reactor was ever built in a large American city.

It took just a few years to construct reactors in the 1960s, because they were relatively small. By the end of 1970, a total of 19 reactors were in operation, with hundreds more scheduled for construction. President Richard Nixon predicted that by the end of the 20th century, one thousand reactors would be operating in the country.

But Nixon's prediction would fall well short. As reactors became larger, the regulatory and construction processes took longer to complete. Ten to fifteen years would often be the time span between the announcement of plans to build a reactor and completion. As construction took long than expected, the bill for reactors mounted; in today's dollars, the cost of building a single reactor is $2 billion or higher. Banks financing reactor projects became impatient, as they waited decades for utilities to generate electricity and income to pay back their loans.

Aside from sky-high costs, the other problem with reactors was safety. In 1966, an accident occurred at the Fermi 1 reactor in southeastern Michigan. Part of the reactor's core melted, and large amounts of radioactivity built up in the containment building. Although the Detroit Edison Company claimed that no radiation was released into the environment, they closed the reactor for four years – and closed it permanently in 1972. In 1975, another accident took place at the Browns Ferry reactor in northern Alabama. Workers sealing a leak with foam rubber held up a lighted candle in a tight space, and accidentally ignited the foam rubber. The roaring fire spread rapidly throughout the plant and damaged a number of safety systems at Browns Ferry. The plant closed for the next 18 months to repair the damage and ensure that all systems were working. Again, the utility claimed that no radiation escaped from the reactor into the air.

These accidents were not the only health threat to the public. Reactors routinely emitted radioactivity into the air. Some of this was accidental, but some was simply a condition of running a reactor. Various safety features reduced the emission doses; the splitting of uranium atoms was controlled, vs. uncontrolled in an atomic bomb; the reactor core was covered with a seal known as cladding; and the core was kept in a containment building. But still it was necessary to emit radioactivity. Each reactor had a stack, which looked somewhat like a smokestack, through which the deadly chemicals passed. In addition, radioactive waste water built up in reactors, and had to be periodically dumped into outside locations.

The AEC responded by setting permissible limits of radioactivity released and present in the environment. It required that each utility report on how much was being emitted and getting into the local environment. But as long as the regulations were met, no further actions were taken. These low doses were presumed to be harmless, and no health studies were done.

Public health departments kept few statistics on health, especially infant and child health, in the 1950s and 1960s, much less than what is collected today. One of the few indicators was infant mortality, or the percent of babies who died before their first birthday. With 98% of children surviving, and with nuclear reactors often located in rural areas (30 miles from large cities) the number of infant deaths among infants exposed to the greatest levels of emissions was often low.

One exception was Peekskill NY, a New York City suburb with a population of about 19,000. After failing to get approval to build a nuclear reactor in the heart of New York City, Consolidated Edison selected Indian Point, a site just two miles from downtown Peekskill. The reactor began operations on August 2, 1962, and reached full capacity on January 1, 1963. The number of Peekskill infants who died between 1960-62 (as the reactor was being built) and 1963-65 (as it operated and emitted radioactivity) soared from 28 to 49, a rise of 72%. This shocking figure went unnoticed by state and local health officials.

The infant death rate is one way to track radiation health risks - but the best way is childhood cancer. Unfortunately, no professional studies were conducted as reactors began operating. More unfortunately, Connecticut was the only state with a reliable registry of cancer cases in the 1960s, joined by Iowa in the 1970s, so a through review of whether more children near nuclear plants developed cancer after they began emitting radioactivity is not possible. But the sparse data from these states suggest that problems were occurring.

In Connecticut, the Haddam Neck reactor started in July 1967, followed by the Millstone 1 reactor in October 1970. The rate of childhood cancer, especially leukemia, had been decreasing in the mid and late 1960s, after the Test Ban Treaty reduced fallout levels in Connecticut and elsewhere. But things changed in a hurry. The number of new leukemia cases in children under age five more than tripled from 1968 to 1971; the number of yearly cases jumped from 7 to 10 to 17 to 25, falling only slightly to 23. The 25 cases in 1971 were the most ever in Connecticut for a single year, with the exception of 1964.

Was it possible that the two new reactors were causing children all across the state to develop leukemia? After all, Connecticut was a small state, and the two reactors were among the largest built to date. Nobody checked out this possibility, until 1990 – a full 33 years since the first reactor began operating - when Senator Edward Kennedy demanded that the federal government study cancer rates near U.S. nuclear plants. The National Cancer Institute responded to Kennedy by producing three thick volumes of data. Most of the report analyzes data on cancer deaths, not cases. But the information on cancer cases in Connecticut and Iowa show a strong connection between reactor startup and cancer in local children.

For children age 0-19, cancer incidence in the reactor's home county is 10% below the state rate before the reactor starts up – and 7% above the state after startup. Increases occurred in all four counties studied, for leukemia and for all other cancers. Because hundreds of cancer cases are involved, this increase is statistically significant.

Years Studied				% Local is +/- State		
Reactor	County	Bef. Start	Aft. Start	Bef. Start	Aft. Start	% Ch.
Haddam Neck	Middlesex CT	'50-'67	'68-'84	-14	-3	+11
Millstone	New London CT	'50-'70	'71-'84	-12	+1	+13
Duane Arnold	Benton/Linn IA	'69-'74	'73-84	+7	+28	+21
Fort Calhoun	Harrison IA	'69-'73	'74-84	-47	+3	+50
TOTAL				-10	+7	+17
Leukemia				+4	+26	+22
Other Cancers				-16	+2	+18

In 2006, a medical journal article took the National Cancer Institute study and examined deaths in children under age ten living near nuclear plants. The study found a distinct pattern in which the death rate was roughly equal to the U.S. average during the first five years after the reactor began operating. But years 6-10 after startup were different; childhood cancer death rates near reactors were nearly 20% greater, covering nearly 600 deaths. A review of childhood cancer near newer nuclear plants found a 15% jump. With tens of millions of Americans living near nuclear plants, this finding is startling.

The rosy future of nuclear power reactors foreseen by government and industry fell apart in the 1970s. The large cost overruns already mentioned, the accidents at places at Fermi and Browns Ferry, and the questions about safety being raised by people like the activist Ralph Nader dissuaded utilities from ordering reactors, and banks from financing them. Hundreds of reactor orders were cancelled. Only a few orders occurred in the 1970s, the last one in 1978. The 1000 reactors predicted by Nixon was never approached; a total of 128 reactors were eventually built. Closings kept this total to never more than 111, and it has been 104 since 1998. In the early 2000s, about 20% of U.S. electricity was produced by nuclear reactors.

The health concerns by Americans posed by nuclear reactors took a sharp turn at a plant on the Susquehanna River in Pennsylvania. Early on the morning of March 28, 1979, maintenance workers at the Three Mile Island plant noticed a clog in one of the pipes at reactor unit 2, which had only been in operation for a few months. Clogs of this type were routine.

But what happened next was anything but routine. The maintenance crew accidentally cut off the cooling water that was constantly needed to keep the reactor core from melting. But without cooling water, the core did just that. The next three days were nightmarish, as industry and government nuclear workers struggled against the accident. It was finally averted, but only after half the core melted. The stricken reactor was permanently disabled.

Panic hit south central Pennsylvania. Thousands of local residents jumped in their cars and fled the area, as officials remained silent. Finally, on the morning of March 30 (over 48 hours after the accident began) Governor Richard Thornburgh issued a recommendation that all pregnant women and children under age five evacuate the area.

Radiation was emitted into the air, but it was unclear just how much, since the existing monitoring systems were unprepared for an event of this magnitude. The Nuclear Regulatory Commission asserted that 14 curies of radioactive particles (with a half life of at least 8 days, which probably would get into the diet and body) were released, more than virtually any reactor had at one time. In addition, 9972 curies of fission and activation gases were released into the air, also a record. Some believed that these levels were understated, and the release was much greater.

Did Three Mile Island harm people? The government, beginning with President Jimmy Carter, who rushed to the site during the accident, assured the public that "nobody died at Three Mile Island." Some medical journal articles estimated that just one or two people would be expected to develop cancer from the meltdown. Other articles ignored the medical effects of radiation, and chose to study psychological effects of the disaster.

But multiple anecdotes were reported. Citizens smelled a foul odor. Infants and elderly felt sick to their stomach and headachy. An unusually high number of local animals developed cancer. Failures were reported in local crops.

And statistics of local humans followed. Children had it worst.

- In Dauphin County, where the reactor was located, the death rate among infants less than one month rose 54% from 1978 to 1979

- In the five years following the accident, the number of children under age 15 living within ten miles of the plant diagnosed with cancer rose from 34 to 47

- The cancer death rate for children under age ten in Dauphin, Lancaster, and York Counties, which was 24% below the U.S. rate in the 1970s, quickly rose to 29% above in the early 1980s

Three Mile Island woke up a nation that had only had modest concerns about nuclear reactors. Almost overnight, polls showed that Americans who feared nuclear power soared. The fear came was spread by media coverage of the accident, along with the recently-released film The China Syndrome starring Jane Fonda, Jack Lemmon, and Michael Douglas, about an accident at a nuclear reactor. Protests sprang up quickly; in May a rally in Washington DC against the proliferation of nuclear power drew 65,000, and later that year, a rally in New York City drew 200,000. Orders for new reactors, which had been dropping in the 1970s, stopped entirely.

On the heels of Three Mile Island, another, much more serious nuclear accident occurred that woke people up to the dangers of nuclear reactors to people – especially children. On April 26, 1986, operators of the Chernobyl nuclear power plant performed an experiment that turned out to be highly reckless. They purposely reduced power to the plant's reactor #4, but in doing so stopped the flow of steam to generators, causing several powerful explosions. The 2000-ton roof of reactor 4 blew completely off, fires blazed throughout the plant, and massive amounts of radioactive gases and particles spewed out to the area, Europe, and the world. Radioactivity was not only breathed, but consumed in food and water.

The damage was so enormous, that 20 years later, the toll is still rising. Some believe that in the end, hundreds of thousands, even millions will suffer from Chernobyl-related diseases. Workers who bravely put out the radioactive fires suffered agonizing deaths from radiation poisoning. The area was evacuated, leaving a permanent ghost town surrounding Chernobyl.

The cloud of fallout from Chernobyl was blasted high into the atmosphere, and began a trek around the world. Scientists monitored one path it took throughout Europe. Another path went directly over the North Pole and entered North America. Beginning May 5, the cloud hovered over the United States, and was brought to earth by rainfall. The greatest precipitation was in the Pacific northwest.

The Environmental Protection Agency measured how much Chernobyl fallout entered the diet, and came up with surprising results. Average levels of Iodine-131 in pasteurized milk were typically 2-3 picocuries (a measure of radioactivity) per liter of milk. But from May 6 until the end of June, levels jumped about three times normal. Places like Boise Idaho, Spokane Washington and Helena Montana averaged 71.0, 42.0 and 30.8, with the highest reading of 136 occurring in Spokane. Conversely, areas with little rainfall were not greatly affected. Tampa Florida, Austin Texas and Wilmington Delaware averaged 2.6, 4.6, and 5.3, respectively. The U.S. government made no effort to caution Americans about contamination in the food supply.

Unfortunately, we will never know the exact toll of Chernobyl. Health professionals and scientists failed to measure doses to local bodies, and did a substandard job of measuring disease trends. But any denial that the toll from the disaster was staggering fell flat when photos of babies with deformities began to circulate around the world. Some were taken abroad to places like the U.S. and Israel for treatment. Anecdotes of large numbers of Soviet children suffering from asthma, pneumonia, and other immune-related diseases circulated.

One scientific advance that came out of Chernobyl occurred just several years after the accident. Medical journals began publishing articles showing a skyrocketing rate of thyroid cancer in local children. In Belarus, just downwind from the reactor, only two children under age 15 were diagnosed with thyroid cancer in 1986, the year of the accident, followed by annual totals of 4, 5, and 6. But beginning in 1990, the numbers leaped to 29 and 55. The average total in the late 1980s in the Ukraine was eight; but this was followed by 26, 22, 48, and 42. Thyroid cancer in children was virtually unheard of before Chernobyl – but the fact that fallout from the accident contained high levels of radioactive iodine, which attacks the thyroid gland, made this ugly trend all too real.

The late 1990s produced discoveries that babies born in 1986 and 1987, who were most likely to suffer most from Chernobyl fallout, were harmed. Rates of leukemia diagnosed in a baby's first year, also a rare occurrence, was 48% greater for births in those two years in West Germany. In Greece, the excess was 160%. And in the United States, 5000-8000 miles from Chernobyl, the excess was 30%.

Thyroid cancer in children and leukemia in infants exposed to Chernobyl radiation was significant. For the first time, hard proof existed that children could develop cancer from early-life exposures to reactor emissions – not 20 or 30 years later, but quickly (4 years in the case of thyroid cancer, and 1 year for leukemia). While levels of fallout from Chernobyl were much higher than any U.S. reactor had emitted, the question was freshly raised: do regular releases from U.S. reactors give children cancer?

Another child health legacy of Chernobyl was that it resurrected the study of Strontium-90 in baby teeth. Largely abandoned after the end of above-ground bomb testing in the 1960s, researchers in Germany, Greece, and the Ukraine examined Sr-90 levels in teeth, and found uniformly that levels were much higher in children born after 1986, compared to those born earlier. The question of whether Sr-90 was linked to risk of cancer or other diseases in children was ignored, however.

CHAPTER 8
U.S. REACTORS CAUSE CHILD HEALTH CONCERNS

Even though orders for new reactors in the U.S. ended after Three Mile Island, and hundreds more planned reactors were scrapped, utilities continued to start up new reactors through the 1980s. By 1990, the number of reactors reached a peak of 111, which produced 20% of the nation's electricity. (Today's figures are 104 reactors and 19% of electricity).

How much radiation reactors were emitting into the environment was pretty much a routine administrative issue. Utilities complied with federal law and made measurements of emissions and levels in the air, water, soil, and milk. No monitoring of radiation in baby teeth or other body organs were done.

Were there any health risks from these emissions? Were children living near nuclear plants more likely to develop cancer? In the first decades that U.S. reactors operated, these were pretty much moot questions, as they just weren't studied.

Perhaps researchers didn't take reactors seriously enough. After all, these weren't atomic weapons, they were atomic energy producers – the "peaceful atom." Perhaps the much lower releases from reactors, compared to bomb tests, into the environment was a factor. Perhaps it was just inertia – this topic had never been studied before. Perhaps it was a lack of public pressure to make these discoveries. Or perhaps the pressure from industry and government to not find out any unpleasant facts was a reason; no voluntary grants from the National Institutes for Health would ever be made to study cancer near reactors.

Health researchers didn't even have a good count of cancer rates among American children. With treatments so advanced, and death rates dropping rapidly, it was incidence rates, or new cases, that became more meaningful. As the years passed, several governments began cancer registries, and in 1973 a national system of cancer registries was formed as part of President Nixon's War on Cancer. Nine states and cities, representing about 10% of the U.S. population, made up this system, called SEER (Surveillance Epidemiology and End Results).

In 1973, the first year for which data are available, the U.S. (SEER) cancer incidence for children under age 15 was 12.7 per 100,000. For much of the next decade, the rate changed little. But after 1984, the rate jumped, first surpassing 14 in 1985 and 15 in 1991. A discussion began over what was causing this increase.

But radiation exposure from nuclear reactors was slow to come into the picture. As late as 1988, only one medical journal study had been published on child cancers near U.S. nuclear reactors. James Enstrom, a public health professor at UCLA, examined death rates near the San Onofre reactor south of Los Angeles, and found no rise in child leukemia deaths after the reactor started. The article was quickly countered by a letter from Carl Johnson, a health official in Colorado who had studied cancer near the Rocky Flats plant near Denver, where plutonium triggers for nuclear weapons had been made. Johnson pointed out that cases, not deaths, were the best means of tracking any impact of reactors. He revealed that only 8 cases of cancer in nine years before the reactor opened were diagnosed in children 0-19 within 25 miles of the plant. In the five year period 1974-1978, however, with the reactor operating at full power, there were 17 cases. But further studies of this area, or those near other reactors, were not made.

The dry spell of studies began to end. Researchers were publishing papers showing high child cancer rates near European reactors. The Three Mile Island accident spurred study of local cancer rates. No articles were published in medical journals until 1990, when a team from Columbia University found that cancer cases in local residents less than 25 years old rose from 34 to 47 in the first five years after the accident. The Columbia group also found that local cancer in children under 15 was more than double the expected rate. But they concluded that the accident had not caused the cancer – rather, that background radiation found in rocks, soil, and air were the likely cause.

In 1988, Senator Edward Kennedy finally brought the issue of cancer near nuclear reactors to the national spotlight. Kennedy, who had a long interest in health issues, ordered the National Cancer Institute to conduct a comprehensive study of cancer near nuclear reactors. Two years later, the NCI released its study.

Similar to what Enstrom and Johnson had found just several years earlier, the death rates for children living near reactors did not show any unusual patterns – but incidence rates near Connecticut and Iowa reactors did. Lead

NCI researcher Seymour Jablon acknowledged in his paper a significant rise in leukemia incidence among Connecticut and Iowa children age 0-9 living near reactors – the only acknowledgment made that reactors were linked with cancer. It wasn't much, but a start, an admission from the government that children developed cancer from reactors.

With limited information from the research community, it was a series of grass roots movements that brought the health risks of living near nuclear reactors, especially for children, to the public eye. And it was in the northeast U.S. that these movements were most pronounced. The northeast had a denser concentration of reactors than any other part of the country, many of them older reactors. And with large population centers like New York, Philadelphia, and Washington, millions of people living in the region were close to at least one reactor.

New Jersey was one of the hotbed areas for the movement to understand health risks of nuclear reactors. This small state, with over 8 million residents, is flanked by New York City and Philadelphia. It has four reactors; the one at Oyster Creek, on the Atlantic Ocean, was the oldest of the 104 U.S. reactors still operating in 2006. Salem/Hope Creek, in the southern part of the state, was one of just two U.S. nuclear plants with three reactors (all others have one or two). The state might have had more reactors, but official orders for four additional ones and plans for an additional six were cancelled in the 1970s.

Health concerns about Oyster Creek were galvanized in 1996, when the Newark Star-Ledger reported an unusually high number of children with cancer in the town of Toms River. The town was located just nine miles downwind (north) of Oyster Creek, and was the home of two other polluting industries, Union Carbide and Ciba-Geigy. From 1979 to 1994, a total of 90 children in Toms River were diagnosed with cancer, significantly higher than the 67 that would be expected if the town rate equaled the state rate.

The reaction of families of stricken children and local citizens in general gave Toms River national attention. Particular attention was focused on environmental factors that may have caused the high rates, and suddenly the aging reactor at Oyster Creek found itself under public scrutiny. The extensive media coverage of the cluster forced federal and state health officials review on environmental causes of the cluster. After nearly six years the $10 million study was released in December 2001. The government found a potential link between leukemia in girls diagnosed before age five if their mother had drank contaminated water while pregnant – but found no other links other than this narrow one, and cautioned that even this one link was not conclusive.

As for Oyster Creek, the report found no link between the reactor's emissions and the childhood cancer cluster. It made the point that actual emissions were far less than the federally-permitted levels, and estimated that emissions would cause one extra cancer death for every BILLION people.

The story of the baby tooth study in New Jersey will be covered in detail in Chapter 10.

Another nuclear plant that made headlines in the 1990s, with concerns over child health at its epicenter was Millstone. The plant was located in southeastern Connecticut, on the Long Island Sound, in the town of Waterford. It was home to three reactors, which started in 1970, 1975, and 1986. Millstone was one of the worst polluters among U.S. nuclear plants; its lifetime airborne emissions ranks third, behind Oyster Creek and Dresden in Illinois.

The clamor over Millstone in the 1990s began early in the decade when the NCI released its report on cancer near nuclear plants. Although rates of many types of cancer rose near reactors after startup, the only one that NCI felt compelled to report as significant was the large increase in childhood leukemia in New London County after the first Millstone reactor began operating.

If the NCI researchers had probed closer, they would have noticed that it wasn't just childhood leukemia that was rising near Millstone. Incidence rates for all cancers in New London County rose faster than the state for all age groups. Incidence of leukemia, thyroid cancer, and bone cancer, which all are closely linked with radiation exposure, were all up. But it was child cancer that was rose most dramatically. New London County, which had levels of child cancer incidence and deaths 12% below the state and nation before Millstone opened, were now 3% and 9% higher, respectively.

The year 1995 meant trouble for Millstone. In August, senior nuclear engineer George Galatis filed a complaint against Northeast Utilities, which ran the plant, for incompetent management practices. Galatis charged that many unsafe procedures were being followed at the plant, and that the safety of the workers and public were at risk. He had brought these complaints to both the utility and the NRC for several years and had gotten nowhere.

Managers at Northeast Utilities denied the charges. Then they formed committees to study the issues but did nothing about it. Galatis reported problems to the NRC; but when he did so, the utility got tough; it downgraded his performance evaluation, and his personnel file was sent to the company legal team. The NRC, meanwhile, denied the Galatis motion – since it had been aware of the situation for nearly a decade. Finally Galatis filed a petition and the news filled the media.

Public hearings followed, and a culture of harassment of "whistle blowers" along with lies and deceitful practices was exposed. Galatis hadn't been the only worker who knew about the safety problems. The corporate structure, along with ineffective regulators, came out as the bad guy. In Galatis' words:

> "At Northeast (Utilities), people are the biggest safety problem. Not the guys in the engine room. The guys who drive the boat."

In March 4, 1996, a Time magazine cover story on Millstone hit the stands. With a photo of Galatis photo on the cover, accompanied by the words 'Blowing the Whistle on Nuclear Safety" the sordid story of Millstone was made public to millions. Northeast Utilities hurriedly shut Millstone reactors 2 and 3 (unit 1 had been closed the previous fall). In the next several years, with the plant producing no electricity, a $1 billion alteration of safety and management procedures took place. The NRC fined the utility $2.1 million, a record. The company pleaded guilty to federal crimes and paid another $10 million in fines.

Millstone 1 was closed permanently, and units 2 and 3 were only re-started in July of 1999 and 1998, respectively. Northeast also shut the Connecticut Yankee reactor in 1996, leaving the state with no nuclear source of electricity. But the state's residents did not experience any unusual blackouts, nor did electric bills skyrocket, during this time.

During the troubled times, the financial health of Northeast Utilities plunged, as the company teetered on the brink of bankruptcy. Eventually it sold Millstone to a larger corporation, Dominion Nuclear of Richmond VA.

But the medical health of local residents, the youngest residents, actually improved when the reactors weren't operating.

In 1994 and 1995, the last two years in which all three Millstone reactors were operating, 85 local infants died before their first birthday. ("Local" means infants from New London county, plus Kent and Washington counties in Rhode Island, which are directly east/downwind of Millstone within 30 miles). In 1996 and 1997, when the plant was closed, the number of infant deaths plunged to 63; in the next two years, when Millstone 2 and 3 gradually resumed operations, the number went to 61. But in 2000-01 and 2002-03, with the two reactors operating over 90% of the time, infant deaths soared again, to 72 and 80, respectively. A similar pattern was followed for deaths to children age 1-9. Although the turnaround was never mentioned by health officials in either state, such a dramatic turnaround might well represent turning Millstone "on" and "off."

Period	Reactors Operating	Infant Deaths
1994-95	3	85
1996-97	0	63
1998-99	1-2	61
2000-01	2	72
2002-03	2	80

Another area in the northeast near a nuclear reactor that featured a battle over child health took place in Long Island. In 1950, the Brookhaven National Laboratory, in the eastern part of the island, about 60 miles from New York City, began operating. Brookhaven was not a nuclear power plant, but a research laboratory that studied various uses of the atom other than warfare. It was not run by a private utility company, but by the U.S. government, who subcontracted the job to a group of Ivy League scientists.

When Brookhaven opened in 1950, the population of Suffolk County, the eastern portion of Long Island was just 667,000. Farms that produced potatoes and other crops still dominated the landscape. Brookhaven had the appearance of a feudal manor when it opened, and it operated in just that way. The Ivy League scientists had little to do with the small town folks in the surrounding communities. But by the 1980s, the population of Suffolk County had doubled, as more people moved from the city to more distant suburbs. Brookhaven was now in the midst of suburban sprawl, and a growing public sensitivity to environmental and health issues.

In the late 1980s, Long Island women became increasingly aware that breast cancer was occurring more frequently. The disease was rising in all parts of the U.S., but appeared to be more common on Long Island. This was puzzling to many. Long Island was a nice place to live. People were better educated, lived in nicer housing, and had better jobs than elsewhere. More importantly, Long Island wasn't fouled by the polluted air of the big cities – but instead of a lower cancer rate, people suspected a higher one.

Their suspicions were correct. In the early 1950s, the breast cancer death rate for white women in Suffolk County was slightly below the U.S. average. But the rate soared 40% by the 1980s, while the national rate didn't change at all. Nearly 300 Suffolk County women died of the disease each year. The rate was high for young women, middle age women, and the elderly. Local residents, with considerable financial clout, got the ear of the politicians rather easily. In 1993 Congress authorized the Long Island Breast Cancer Study Project, and poured millions of dollars into research to find what was causing breast cancer rates to rise. Brookhaven was not considered by study researchers, who were mostly from Columbia University.

Brookhaven had emitted considerable levels of radiation and other chemicals into the local environment, but their practices went virtually unchecked until the late 1980s, when it was designated as a Superfund site. In the mid-1990s, citizens and media brought these practices to the public's attention, and things began to go downhill fast for the lab. Some of the findings were:

- Leaks of radioactive tritium from the waste pools for 12 years were not fixed
- Local residents with cancer sued Associated Universities and the Energy Department
- The Energy Department fired Associated Universities for incompetence
- High levels of Strontium-90 and other chemicals were found in groundwater at BNL

In 1996, as the battle over Brookhaven raged, Dr. Jay Gould got the idea to form a citizens group to fight for public accountability – and ultimately, closure of the two reactors still operating. Gould was a retired economic statistician from New York City who had a summer home in Long Island. A decade earlier, he had founded the Radiation and Public Health Project, a group of scientists and health professionals, to do research on the cancer risks of nuclear reactors. Now Gould saw the need to add a local citizens group dedicated to the radiation health issue. The result was Standing for Truth About Radiation, or the STAR Foundation.

STAR was no ordinary grassroots group. It drew from the sector of affluent, politically savvy people who lived in Long Island, including actor Alec Baldwin and model Christie Brinkley. Through a blitz of public education and lobbying, efforts by STAR persuaded numerous politicians such as Senator Alfonse D'Amato to call for greater accountability from BNL, and eventually, its closing. And STAR was successful; the Energy Department closed the last two Brookhaven reactors in 1996 and 1999, and began the long, expensive cleanup process.

Local childhood cancer played a significant role in the campaign over Brookhaven, much of it spearheaded by Randy Snell. A banker, Snell lived in Manorville, an upscale suburb just four miles from Brookhaven, with his wife and four daughters. One day in 1996, Snell's life changed forever when his four year old daughter Lauren was diagnosed with rhabdomyosarcoma, a disease so obscure that many take a while to learn its pronunciation. Rhabdo is a soft tissue cancer that is most common in children.

Snell and his wife went through the agonizing ritual that all parents of children with cancer do, a series of visits to the doctor and the hospital for tests and treatments. Lauren, whose cancer was found in her mouth, recovered from the ordeal and survived. And as she began to recover, Snell turned his thoughts from "will she live?" to "why did this happen?" As he recalled:

> "When my daughter was suffering from the disease, one day she grabbed me around the neck and asked 'Why, daddy, why?' I was determined to find out, and I discovered that the only cause of this disease is low-level radiation."

Snell found that indeed, researchers had linked radiation exposure to rhabdo. Like Alice Stewart had done 40 years earlier, X-rays during pregnancy doubled the chance that the baby would develop rhabdo during childhood. No other reason for rhabdo had been clearly identified. Snell also discovered just by talking to others in hospital waiting rooms and around the community that there were 19 cases of childhood rhabdo in the small portion of Long Island near Brookhaven – a number about 22 times what would normally be expected. The discovery galvanized Snell to action. "I decided to find out why this area was dripping with cancers," he said.

The response he got from officials was one of denial. After being notified, New York State Department of Health official Claire Pospisial issued a cold thumbs-down statement:

> "Based upon the information we have from the state cancer registry, we don't believe that there is an unusual incidence or an increase in the number of cases of rhabdomyosarcoma."

But the STAR Foundation took up Snell's cause. Led by Christie Brinkley, STAR lobbied for a full investigation into the rhabdo cluster. Brinkley told Suffolk County legislators it was "your job and your responsibility to protect our community." In August 2000, legislature passed a law mandating a special rhabdo task force, which met periodically for the next several years. But the committee was slowed by the leadership of the county health department, which was in no hurry to find a cause. The committee disbanded without finding a link between rhabdo and radiation exposure from Brookhaven.

It turns out that Long Island had high rates in children not just of rhabdo, but of all cancers. From 1997-2001, a total of 720 Long Islanders under age 20 were diagnosed with cancer, which translated to a rate 21% above the national average, and higher than almost all large counties in New York state. But no acknowledgement from the health establishment or Brookhaven was ever made of this fact. More amazingly, the Long Island Breast Cancer Study concluded in 2002 – after a decade and $30 million in federal tax dollars – and found no connection with any form of pollution (radiation from Brookhaven was not even considered as a factor). The end of the breast cancer study brought with it the assertion by some that there had NEVER BEEN an epidemic in the first place. The New York Times, which had supported the study, ran an editorial entitled "Breast Cancer Mythology on Long Island" that said

> "The search for environmental causes for a supposed breast cancer epidemic on Long Island is beginning to look like a wild goose chase."

Dr. Deborah Winn of the National Cancer Institute made a statement about the Long Island breast cancer epidemic: "I don't think it is reflective of any reality. I don't know where it comes from. It's myths." But many were still unconvinced, and unhappy with the study.

The Brookhaven leadership also made no admission that the reactors had harmed Long Islanders. In 2003, lab director Dr. Praveen Chaudhari commented on the closing of Brookhaven reactors.

> "If I was a neighbor of Brookhaven, not knowing what was going on and suddenly learning that something will be coming my way in my drinking water, or in my soil, I'd worry about it too. And I might respond in a certain way. But the newspapers got involved, and they had a story to write. The net result was that it all spiraled out of proportion."

Another nuclear plant in which childhood cancer worries became more prominent in the 1990s was a famous (or infamous) name in U.S. history – Three Mile Island. The 1979 accident caused the permanent closing of the stricken reactor #2, and the temporary closing of the other reactor #1, which did not re-start for nearly seven years. The health effects first were documented as anecdotes of local citizens who developed cancer soon after the meltdown. Some of these were children. As we observed in the last chapter, cancer cases in persons under age 25 living within ten miles of Three Mile Island jumped 38% (from 34 to 47) in the first five years after the accident.

GPU, the utility that operated the plant, quickly set up a fund and eventually paid over $30 million to settle claims from the accident – without admitting any harm caused by radiation. Even with this, many people suffering from cancer, including children, decided to take their case to court. Naturally, it was a long and laborious task, but nearly two decades after the meltdown, the case made it to federal court on behalf of 2,000 local citizens. But quickly, judge Sylvia Rambo dismissed the case. Rambo threw out the testimony of several expert witnesses that lawyers for the citizens had hoped would prove the case that radiation from the accident had caused cancer. The decision ended any chance that the utility would be held officially accountable for radiation-induced damage.

Over a quarter-century after the Three Mile Island accident, many still hold that many were damaged from radioactive releases. Local resident Alice

Deimier, who lost a 6 year old son to cancer soon after the accident, said:
> "He was a normal, healthy boy before the accident… I still blame Three Mile Island."

While there will probably never be complete agreement on how much damage was caused, considerable evidence exists that many, especially children, were harmed. In Dauphin County (where the plant is located) and Lebanon County (adjacent to the east/downwind direction), there were 246 children under age twenty diagnosed with cancer from 1985-1997, a rate 26% above the state and nation. (The state cancer registry only began collecting data in 1985). Cancer mortality in the two counties was even worse, with a rate 39% above the U.S. from 1980-2003 (120 deaths).

One problem with the dismissed Three Mile Island law suit was that there was no evidence of how much radioactivity from the reactor had entered the bodies of local residents. This fact was not lost on at least one curious observer.

CHAPTER 9
THE TOOTH FAIRY PROJECT CHALLENGES U.S. REACTORS

In 1996, Jay Gould read accounts of Judge Rambo's dismissal of the Three Mile Island law suit with vivid interest. Gould was a retired economic statistician from New York City. He had received his PhD from Columbia and had a very successful career as an expert witness in anti-trust actions. In his last case, Gould had represented the Westinghouse corporation; as he did background reading, he learned that Westinghouse was one of two companies (along with General Electric) that had designed the great majority of nuclear reactors in the U.S.

Gould soon made the acquaintance of Dr. Ernest Sternglass, a physicist. Sternglass had worked at Westinghouse Laboratories in the 1950s and 1960s before becoming a professor of physics and public health at the University of Pittsburgh. Retired as well, Sternglass had moved to New York City so his wife Marilyn could take a job at the City University of New York. They moved into an apartment on Manhattan's Upper West Side, which was (unbeknownst to him at the time) just ten blocks from where Gould lived with his wife Jane.

One night, Gould wanted to hear Sternglass give a talk. He wasn't feeling well, but pushed himself to go and introduce himself to the physicist. Gould could not have imagined what awaited him. Sternglass gave a fiery talk about the long history of man-made radioactivity in the U.S., first from atomic bomb tests and then from nuclear reactors. Unlike most physicists, Sternglass was not content with just the technical counting of radioactivity levels. Because both of his parents had been physicians, he had always been interested in health and medicine – and thus was eager to know the health effects of radiation exposure.

In 1969, Sternglass had shocked the nation when he published an article in Esquire magazine entitled "The Death of All Children." Sternglass estimated that 375,000 American infants had died as a result of fallout from above-ground atomic bomb tests. He wrote:

> "Infant mortality had shown a steady decline in the period 1935-1950; but beginning with the Nevada tests in 1951 and continuing until just after the test ban in 1963, the rate suddenly leveled off in the U.S."

In the article, Sternglass singled out the actions of Strontium-90 on human reproductive cells as backing for his theory of harm to infants. He referred to the buildup of Sr-90 bodies of American children from the "so-called baby-tooth survey" in St. Louis. Sternglass was roundly criticized for being an "alarmist", mostly by government and industry officials – although to this day, no other plausible explanation for the trend in infant mortality has ever been made.

Gould and Sternglass began to correspond, visiting each other frequently. Soon Gould hatched the idea for an independent group of professionals dedicated to studying health effects of radioactivity from bombs and reactors. The government wasn't going to examine the topic honestly, Gould reasoned, as it would be unlikely to admit that its bomb program had harmed Americans. Academic researchers could do the work, but many university-based health professionals relied heavily on government funds and didn't want to risk losing funds by making conclusions that put the finger on the bomb program. Any solid research had to come from independent sources. Gould, a wealthy man, would fund the group himself. He named the effort the Radiation and Public Health Project (RPHP), and Sternglass became the chief scientist.

RPHP got off to a solid start. Gould published two books, entitled Deadly Deceit and The Enemy Within, that were chock full of statistical evidence that Americans had been harmed by bombs and reactors. Gould and Sternglass, along with Joseph Mangano, a public health administrator who had taken an interest in the work and joined the group, wrote several articles in medical journals as well. Bill McDonnell joined the group as the data and financial manager. Gould also hit upon the idea for a local advocacy group to work with RPHP, which turned into the STAR Foundation on Long Island.

Gould himself was a modest man, and RPHP reflected it. He declined to set up an office for the group, opting instead for each member to work from their home office. Gould and Sternglass did not set any pre-conceived agenda for the group, preferring to encourage free academic thought instead. "I've always believed that if one of gets an idea, and talks it over with the others, we should go with it," explained Gould years later.

In 1996, Gould read the account of the failed Three Mile Island law suit. He had been disturbed by the failure of government researchers to even consider radioactive emissions from Brookhaven as a potential cause of breast cancer on Long Island. Gould realized that for any change in nuclear policy to occur, stronger evidence of radiation damage was needed. He knew that since the Department of Energy ended the study of Strontium-90 in adult bones in 1982, the nation had been without any program that measured radiation in human bodies, especially those who lived near nuclear reactors.

Sternglass remembers that in October 1996, he and Gould discussed these issues. When the St. Louis baby tooth survey was mentioned, Gould had a thought: why not duplicate the study of Sr-90 in baby teeth, replacing bomb fallout with U.S. reactor emissions? Sternglass readily agreed. The Tooth Fairy Project was born.

Only one study of in-body radiation near nuclear reactors had ever been conducted. A group of British scientists had recently studied baby teeth from various distances to the Sellafield reactor in northwest England. The leader of the group, R.G. O'Donnell, had presented results for his master's thesis, and had submitted them to a journal for publication. They found that the closer children lived to Sellafield, the higher the average level of plutonium in baby teeth. But there was no such link with Strontium-90 or all radioactive chemicals emitting alpha particles. Moreover, the British group dismissed the possibility that these levels of radioactivity in teeth could pose a health threat.

The first task for Gould and Sternglass was to find a laboratory to test teeth. Both knew Hari Sharma, a radiochemist from Waterloo, Canada. Gould had recently met Sharma at a conference in Vienna, when Sharma made a presentation observing the 10th anniversary of the Chernobyl accident. "Jay seemed to know all about me" recalls Sharma. "What I had to say, he must have liked it." In late October 1996, Sternglass spoke with Sharma, who agreed to find a machine and determine a procedure to test baby teeth.

Sharma held a PhD in nuclear chemistry from the University of California, and had been doing studies of uranium in urine of nuclear workers when Sternglass called him. Realizing how costly the job would be and how small RPHP was, Sharma graciously agreed to test teeth without any direct compensation paid to him: RPHP would only be billed for the cost of equipment, materials, and lab technician time. Sharma also excited Gould and Sternglass when he informed them that individual teeth could be accurately tested using the most current machines. This was major news, since all other studies of Sr-90 in baby teeth, including St. Louis, had tested teeth in batches. Knowing the Sr-90 level of individual teeth would allow RPHP to set up health studies, i.e. whether children with the highest Sr-90 level are sicker.

Sharma determined that a liquid scintillation counter was the best type of machine for this job. Sharma would first clean the tooth, crush it into a powder, and then separate out any decay or fillings, leaving only the healthy enamel for testing. The powder was dissolved in a liquid solution, and placed into the machine for counting. The amount of Sr-90 was not measured in volume, but in "counts" since the amount of radioactive decay was what was being measured. Sharma determined that to be accurate, each tooth needed to be tested for 400 minutes. Although this upped the cost of testing a single tooth to about $50, Gould and Sternglass readily accepted the plan, in order to obtain the most accurate information possible.

They also accepted Sharma's plan to take a small amount of each tooth and send it to a laboratory for measuring calcium. When both Sr-90 and calcium measurements were made, a ratio of the two – picocuries of Sr-90 per gram of calcium – was possible, just as Rosenthal had done in St. Louis many years earlier. Sharma did a test run on 50 teeth in 1998, and after some slight adjustments, was ready to embark on the study.

The Tooth Fairy Project was first launched on Long Island, where the Brookhaven battle was in full swing and where Gould maintained a summer home. On June 15, 1997, Suffolk county orthodontist Milton Bloch wrote an editorial in the magazine Suffolk Life. Bloch had met with Gould, and the two had taped a half-hour show for cable television. After learning about the large number of rhabdomyosarcoma cases near Brookhaven, Bloch was hooked on the tooth study.

> "On April 21, I watched a remarkable NBC Channel 4 interview with the Theobald family living near BNL, whose seven year old son Jeffrey had been diagnosed with an extremely rare form of cancer called rhabdomyosarcoma. The Theobalds were convinced that BNL was responsible and that they were therefore contributing Jeffrey's baby teeth to a study of its strontium-90 content being done by the non-profit Radiation and Public Health Project (RPHP) headed by Dr. Jay M. Gould… Galvanized by this chilling newscast, and knowing about the great sensitivity of this method of measuring radiation-induced harm, I called Dr. Gould… "

The big boost for the baby tooth study came in 1999. Gould hit upon the idea of sending a mass mailing to Long Island families with young children who were losing baby teeth and thus most likely to have saved a tooth. He obtained an electronic tape of households, with the name and address of parents. In late winter 1999, a mailing of 15,000 letters from actor Alec Baldwin was sent, with a picture of a Tooth Fairy on the envelope. The Baldwin letter was addressed "Dear Parent" but was aimed directly at the well-known issue of cancer on Long Island:

> "I am writing you as someone personally concerned that our high cancer rates may be influenced by radioactive reactor emissions in the greater New York metropolitan area.
> One hypothesis is that these high cancer rates may be largely caused by radioactive leaks and emissions from nuclear reactors… These reactors include Brookhaven National Laboratory on Long Island, Indian Point in New York, Millstone in Connecticut, and Oyster Creek in New Jersey.
> To document a possible radiation/cancer connection, we only need one or two of the baby teeth that your children lose between the ages of 5 and 12."

In May, Baldwin showed up personally to moderate a panel discussion at the Westhampton Beach Performing Arts Center to push the tooth study. He addressed the large crowd by again taking a personal approach, by citing his mother, who had survived breast cancer:

> "I wish I didn't have to be here to organize a group of research scientists, who will tell you about the radiological and chemical contamination we're experiencing on Long Island, where I grew up as well. But my mother is a breast cancer survivor, who has dedicated the second act of her life to working on breast cancer research, and I want to help her find answers."

Baldwin also freely gave his time for interviews. In mid-1999, he explained to one reporter that the reason he was so deeply involved with the radiation health issue was that "it is the most difficult cause I have ever been involved in." He gave a strong answer when asked why he considered the issue so difficult:

> "It's because your opponent – the government – is the most enigmatic.

Or perhaps inscrutable is the better word. When you sit down across from the government, it's hard to find your way. Because the first thing they do is deny, deny, deny that there is a problem. It makes me think of some town in the old west riddled with graft and the sheriff and his boys just say to the townspeople 'Now you all go on home, there's nothing to worry about, we're taking care of it'."

Despite all the promotion, Gould and his colleagues crossed their fingers that the study would be a hit. And it was, beyond anyone's wildest dreams. By June 1999, over 1100 baby teeth had been sent to RPHP, most from Long Island. Another area with considerable tooth donations was central New Jersey, near the Oyster Creek nuclear reactor. Several thousand letters from Baldwin had been sent there as well.

Sharma went to work testing the teeth. Although he had a backlog of over 1000, he could only test 20 per week because of the long period spent on each tooth to make results as accurate as possible. Results of the first several dozen teeth came back, but RPHP waited until several hundred were tested until speaking out.

What they found was shocking. The average concentration of Strontium-90 in baby teeth was about 1.5 picocuries per gram of calcium. When Gould and Sternglass referred to old articles on the St. Louis study, they realized that the 1.5 average was reached for children born in 1956. This was less than the 11.0 figure at the 1963-1964 height of bomb test fallout, but much greater than the 0.2 found for children born in 1950, before bomb testing began in Nevada. And the current teeth were from children born in the late 1980s and early 1990s, long after atmospheric testing had ended. There may have been differences between the RPHP and St. Louis machines, so the results may not have been exactly apples to apples. But RPHP members believed they had a big story – a "second nuclear weapons testing era."

In late summer 1999, with results of 300 teeth in hand, Gould felt confident enough to speak out candidly:

> "The levels look as though they've been taken during the (nuclear weapons) testing years. It just freaked us out when we got to the results."

There were many more teeth to be tested, but the group agreed that the word needed to be spread quickly. Spreading the word could only be done through the media. And the media would be most interested if the group produced a medical journal article. Journals require a "peer review" before publication, involving a review by experts not known to the authors. Often articles are returned for modifications, or rejected outright. The group decided to try the International Journal of Health Services. It had been published since the 1970s and had a number of esteemed health professionals on its editorial board. It seemed to be interested in the radiation health issue, and had published two earlier articles by RPHP members.

The task of writing the article fell to Mangano, who had done all the group's articles in the late 1990s. He knew it had to be technically correct, so he explained the study methods in detail, with the help of Sharma, who provided a technical explanation of how teeth were tested. He knew that statements would need to be supported by other journal articles, and included 62 professional references. The basic results of Sr-90 in teeth were actually straightforward. There were 515 baby teeth, but only the 476 who were born after 1979 were used, since those born earlier probably still had Sr-90 left over from bomb testing. Of the total of 476 teeth in the study, the 38 teeth from Miami FL had the highest average of 2.80, compared to the national average of 1.50.

But the biggest issue was health hazards. Did the group have any evidence that the Strontium-90 was linked with higher disease rates in humans? And if so, which disease? Sternglass had the immediate answer: "childhood cancer." When Mangano asked him what age group should be looked at first, Sternglass had another prompt reply: "As young as possible." And so Mangano scoured his files in search of data on cancer cases diagnosed in children before age five. And since 304 of the 476 teeth were from children who lived in Suffolk County on Long Island, the most significant results would come from this county.

Working quickly, Mangano calculated the average Sr-90 level in baby teeth by birth year, along with cancer incidence age 0-4 by year of diagnosis. He grabbed a sheet of paper and made a rough graph with two lines, one for Sr-90 and one for cancer. He was puzzled when the lines looked very different. When Sr-90 went up, cancer often went down, and vice versa.

But by staring at the raw numbers he noticed something. Sr-90 steadily increased from 1981 to 1986, about 50%, from 1.0 to 1.5 picocuries per gram of calcium, followed by a decline. And cancer incidence steadily increased from 1984 to 1989, also by about 50%, and also followed by a decline. Mangano redrew the graph, but shifted the cancer line by three years. What he produced was quite remarkable. The two lines looked virtually the same. He called Sternglass: could there be a lag of about three years from exposure to cancer diagnosis? "Absolutely" said Sternglass, reciting the numerous studies that had found the same thing. "The fetus is most susceptible to radiation, so we would expect cancer in young children to be the first evidence of adding Strontium-90 to the body."

Mangano whipped the numbers and graph off to Gould, and the statistician quickly called back to say that the "r value was .85," a sophisticated way of saying that the close match in the two lines was statistically significant. The first-ever link between Sr-90 in baby teeth and cancer had been found. And the idea that only a rise of 0.5 picocuries of Sr-90, a very tiny amount, could boost child cancer by 50% was an amazing revelation of the power of even low dose radiation.

After several weeks in which the phone lines between the Gould, Sternglass, and Mangano households were working overtime, the group had its draft article, complete with the Sr-90/cancer graph. Several weeks of proofreading and corrections later, it was sent to the journal. And several weeks later, the good news came in: the article was accepted. The group followed up with two other articles, one of which was written by Dr. Janette Sherman, a Virginia toxicologist who was helping the group. By the fall of 2000, the study had been published in three medical journals, the gold standard of research.

As the articles neared publication, the group had a big decision to make. Sharma was retiring from the University of Waterloo, which meant he could no longer use the Waterloo machines to measure Sr-90. The group needed to find another machine, which was not an inexpensive proposition. They could have found another radiochemist to do the study, but since everybody was pleased with Sharma's work, the decision was made to buy a new machine for Sharma to use. After some shopping, the group decided to buy the Perkin-Elmer 1220-003 liquid scintillation counter, perhaps the most advanced machine in measuring low doses of radioactivity with the greatest precision. The price tag was $75,000, a heavy burden for the small group, but the tooth study was too important.

So in June 2000, after 1303 teeth had been tested, the new Perkin Elmer machine was sent to Sharma's home office and set up for use. The new machine marked a turning point in the study. With the old machine, Sharma had only been able to detect Sr-90 in about 70% of the teeth – even though all contained some amount of the chemical. The new machine could detect more Sr-90, especially if the teeth were cleaned with hydrogen peroxide and not water. But this change meant that the first 1303 teeth could not be compared with teeth tested thereafter, and RPHP would have to maintain two separate data bases. But the group believed it was worth using the new method, and eventually Sr-90 was detected in about 95% of the teeth tested using the new counter, a great improvement.

Collecting teeth was not an easy task. Even the letters sent by Alec Baldwin produced only a 1 or 2 percent return - at a high cost. RPHP members recalled that the St. Louis study relied heavily on volunteers who directly appealed for tooth donations. They encouraged citizens to take charge on tooth collections, sending tooth envelopes and explanatory letters to anyone who requested them. An 800 number was set up for anyone to call in and request envelopes and flyers. Eventually, thousands were given out.

Westchester County, just north of New York City, would provide teeth to RPHP through a combination of mass mailings, citizen outreach, and government support. The Indian Point nuclear plant, located in the northwestern part of the county, had long been a target for anti-nuclear activists, partly because it was located near the most densely populated city in the U.S. And the three reactors at the site had had problems. The Indian Point 1 reactor had closed permanently in 1974 after only 12 years in operation, and thereafter its waste leaked gradually into the Hudson River. Indian Point 3 had been closed for nearly three years in the mid-1990s due to mechanical problems before restarting. And in February 2000, Indian Point 2 experienced the worst-ever accident at the plant. Officials assured that no radiation was released into the air, but the reactor was closed for one year to make repairs.

Perhaps the biggest blow against Indian Point was the terrorist attacks on September 11, 2001. One of the planes that crashed into the World Trade Center had been hijacked soon after its departure from Boston, and flew down the Hudson River towards New York City – directly over Indian Point. The realization that the terrorists could have ordered the plane to crash into the plant with its massive amount of deadly radiation struck fear into many, who organized a crash program to close the plant down. The group Riverkeeper, directed by environmental lawyer Robert F. Kennedy Jr., spent a large proportion of its resources to closing Indian Point after the terrorist attacks.

Even before the September 11 attacks, the Tooth Fairy Project had a great reception in Westchester. Without the benefit of a mass mailing appealing for tooth donations, over 100 teeth from the area near Indian Point were sent to RPHP. Many of the teeth were the result of Margo Schepart's efforts. Schepart, a local teacher and mother of two children, had been interested in environmental issues, but became particularly focused on Indian Point after hearing Gould speak in 1995. When the tooth study began several years later, Schepart saw it as the "perfect vehicle to wake people up to the reality of the health effects of ionizing radiation released by Indian Point."

She took it upon herself to collect teeth by dressing up as the tooth fairy, and going to local events asking for donations.

> "I bought a beautiful purple satin prom gown at Goodwill, attached some wings, and appeared as the Tooth Fairy at many local summer events. I talked to many children and their parents as I distributed collection envelopes and literature about the tooth project. I would frequently wander around the grounds of these events in costume, playing my guitar... From year to year I would see the same families during the summer festivals. They would bring me teeth that they said they had been saving all winter for me."

Results showed that average Sr-90 in the two closest counties to the east (downwind), Westchester and Putnam, had the highest Sr-90 levels in New York state, higher than New York City, higher than Long Island (the home of the Brookhaven lab). Rates of cancer in local children and adolescents were also above the state and nation, even though the area was largely a tony suburban area with relatively few economic and social problems, plus good access to medical care.

RPHP, urged by Baldwin, decided to ask the Westchester County legislature for financial support in late 2000, so more teeth could be collected, making the study more significant. To that point, RPHP had not received a penny from government. Attempts to obtain funds had been squashed by New Jersey governor Christine Whitman (who had line-item vetoed a $75,000 provision to RPHP, saying it was a federal responsibility) and Suffolk County executive Robert Gaffney (who held up a $35,000 provision, claiming RPHP didn't have the facilities and equipment to do the study). This time, the effort would include a famous figure making the pitch for funds, and it would be done in front of the cameras.

On November 2, 2000, Baldwin, Mangano, RPHP Executive Director Jerry Brown, and STAR Executive Director Robert Alvarez made a presentation to the Health Committee of the county legislature. With considerable press there, Baldwin asked for $50,000 in funds to make the tooth study results near Indian Point significant. With numerous press members in attendance, he pointed to the members of the public and said

> "If there are elevated levels of strontium here, you make the call, you make the decision. Do you want to live in the shadow of that kind of thing?"

Several of the legislators spoke out in favor of the study. Chief among them was committee chair Tom Abinanti, who cited his responsibility to protect public health.

> "As locally elected officials, we have to highlight the health hazard that is present in our Westchester community. I have a mandate to protect the people."

The large amount of press that followed gave RPHP the chance to fully air the study and the concerns behind it. In an interview with a local weekly paper, Mangano spoke about the skewed view of preventive health in the U.S.

> "To me, there should be such a frantic attempt at preventing cancer, but we're really not doing it. It's only focused on individuals: 'Stop smoking, Joe. Put more fiber in your diet so you don't get colon cancer.' But when it comes to nuclear reactors, there's silence."

Soon after the Baldwin visit, the Westchester legislature voted solidly to grant RPHP $25,000 to collect and test 250 more local baby teeth. The group was ecstatic; even though politicians in New Jersey and Long Island had kept funds from them, the politicians in Westchester had been won over by Baldwin – or so they thought. Six months after the vote, RPHP was in trouble again, this time from the County Health Department, which had written four long letters in that time. Each of the letters expressed concerns with the study's methods, and each was answered dutifully by Mangano – only to be followed by another letter with more complaints. County Health Director Dr. Joshua Lipsman explained later

> "The Health Department... has brought several serious flaws in the project's scientific methodology to Mr. Mangano's attention. To date, he has not remedied them, thus questioning the validity of the project's research findings."

But this time, RPHP was not going to roll over and give up the funds. Mangano contacted a local newspaper and explained the situation, charging the Health Department with deliberately holding up the funds for political reasons. Several weeks after the article appeared, the Health Department released the money. With the aid of another letter signed by Baldwin to thousands of local parents, RPHP went on to collect and test the 250 local teeth. They found that average Sr-90 from the three counties closest to Indian Point was 36% greater than in the rest of New York State; and that local children born in the late 1990s had Sr-90 levels 56% greater than those born in the late 1980s. Despite the political struggles, and despite the fact that Indian Point continued to operate, the tooth study near Indian Point was a great success.

Early in 2001, just after the Baldwin visit to Westchester County, RPHP set its sights on another area. About 20 miles northwest of Philadelphia stood the Limerick nuclear plant (with two reactors) in the town of Pottstown. The town was also the site of two other polluting industries, a waste landfill and a plastics manufacturing plant. Janette Sherman had visited the area, and found it to be highly polluted and suspected that cancer rates were high, and recommended that RPHP include the Limerick area in its tooth study.

Pushed by the local citizen group Alliance for a Clean Environment (ACE), the Montgomery County Health Department had conducted a study of cancer in the Pottstown area. They found that from 1985-1994, cancer incidence in children under age 20 was 50% greater than the rest of the area. But cynically, because only 33 children were diagnosed in this time, the department dismissed this finding, that "average annual childhood cancer rates for these areas do not differ significantly."

Mangano reviewed the most current statistics, and was astounded, especially by the child cancer situation. In the 1990s, the cancer incidence rate for children under 20 in the greater Pottstown area was 77% greater, nearly double, than the area, state, and nation, based on 40 diagnosed cases. And this time, it WAS statistically significant. But it was not just cancer cases, but cancer deaths, that were high. Cancer mortality in Montgomery County, where Limerick is located, soared 48% from 1984-90 (when Limerick was just beginning to operate) to 1990-2002. But in the same period, the national rate fell 20%. Similar to Westchester County, Montgomery County is one of the most affluent in the nation, and had no obvious risks of cancer.

Mangano's visit to Pottstown in January 2001 was well covered by the local press. Other speakers included the ACE president, a local radiologist, and the Pottstown mayor. Without the benefit of a visit or letter from Baldwin, over 100 teeth were sent to RPHP. During a return visit in November 2003, Mangano announced that the average Sr-90 level near Limerick was the highest of the seven plants in which RPHP had a substantial number of teeth.

Southern Florida became another focal point for the tooth study, for several reasons. Jerry Brown was based in Miami. There were four reactors in the area; the two St. Lucie reactors were near Port St. Lucie and the two Turkey Point reactors were just south of Miami. And starting in the mid-1990s, an unexpectedly large cluster of cancer cases in Port St. Lucie began making the headlines, and local citizens demanded to know causes of the epidemic. The town was located just eight miles from the St. Lucie reactors.

Statistics showed that there was indeed a high child cancer rate in St. Lucie county. In 1981-83, 4 children under age ten living in the county were diagnosed with cancer. By 1996-98, the number had surged to 30. But the surge was more than just one town. An article by Mangano, Sherman, and some medical students in New York City showed cancer incidence age 0-9 near all 14 eastern U.S. nuclear plants were higher than the nation – but the two highest were in St. Lucie/Martin counties (closest to St. Lucie) and Dade county (closest Turkey Point). The data covered the years 1988-1997, with a total of 651 cancer cases in the three counties.

In March 2001, Brown and Sternglass held a press conference in Miami, releasing the initial results of the tooth study and appealing for more tooth donations. The conference was well covered by a number of Florida television stations and newspapers. But news reached beyond Florida, perhaps because of the childhood cancer epidemic. The Associated Press ran a story, and National Public Radio used a brief in its newscast. But the best press came from overseas. The British Broadcasting Company filmed a news story which was broadcast soon after to an audience of about 90 million, including some in the U.S.

Soon after the press conference, Brown was successful in obtaining a grant from the Health Foundation of South Florida; with the funds, RPHP sent out a mass mailing of the Baldwin letter, and received many more teeth. In 2003, another press conference was held to announce the results. Over 500 additional teeth from the state had been tested, most from the areas near the Turkey Point and St. Lucie reactors. Results were similar to other areas; teeth near the reactors had an average Sr-90 level about 45% higher than the rest of Florida, and had risen 36% since the late 1980s.

The public call to find causes of the childhood cancer epidemic in Port St. Lucie – especially environmental causes - forced the county health department to conduct a study. The department examined 561 chemicals, and found no evidence that any of them had contributed to the problem. Incredibly, radiation emitted from the St. Lucie plant was not on this long list, and RPHP continued to press its case that high and rising Sr-90 levels near the plant had contributed to cancer risk in children. But Florida Power and Light, which ran the St. Lucie plant, hotly disputed any responsibility, minimized the effects of radiation exposure, criticized the tooth study, and even denied that local cancer rates were high. Company spokesperson Rachel Scott expressed this blind eye to the many facts;

> "Their (RPHP) claims are false. Cancer levels are not higher in South Florida. The levels of Strontium-90 are not higher in South Florida, according to the Florida Department of Health and the Nuclear Regulatory Commission."

By 2003, the total number of tooth donations neared 4000, close to the 5000 originally envisioned by Gould to make a significant study. At least 100 teeth were from children who lived near any of six nuclear power plants (the Brookhaven research lab made seven). It was time to publish another article, a more comprehensive article than the first three. Again, RPHP was strict with which teeth to include. The 1303 teeth tested on the old machine were excluded. Teeth with too little enamel for an accurate Sr-90 level were excluded. Teeth where the parent didn't specify the residence were excluded. But that still left 2089 teeth tested on the new, more sophisticated machine.

Results were amazingly consistent near each nuclear plant. Average Sr-90 in counties closest to plants were about 30 to 50 percent higher than in other counties in the state. Average Sr-90 began rising in the late 1980s, and by the late 1990s were 35 to 60 percent higher. With the large number of teeth, all results were statistically significant. Mangano submitted an article to the British journal The Science of the Total Environment, which had earlier published articles on Sr-90 in baby teeth from Great Britain, Greece, and the Ukraine. Although the journal's two reviewers were sharply split – one thought it was worthy of publication, the other thought it wasn't – the journal published it in December 2003.

In the days following, the newspaper USA Today published a long story on the Tooth Fairy Project. This was another breakthrough for RPHP, as USA Today had the highest daily circulation (over 2 million) of any U.S. newspaper. The article related RPHPs conclusion that the recent substantial jump in average Sr-90 levels in teeth could only be due to a current source of radiation, and that could only be nuclear reactors. Naturally, quotes from opponents of the study were included, but so was a quote from former Energy Department official Robert Alvarez as not being convinced that RPHP had completely made its case, but "there may be a correlation between strontium-90 in baby teeth and childhood cancers."

CHAPTER 10
THE TOOTH FAIRY PROJECT IN NEW JERSEY

Of all the places where the Tooth Fairy Project made its mark, New Jersey was perhaps the one with the greatest impact.

New Jersey was an inviting target from the beginning. Situated just across the Hudson River from RPHPs home base in New York, it is one of the most densely populated U.S. states, ranking 47th in area but 9th in population. In the early years of the nuclear age, many nuclear reactors were envisioned for New Jersey. Of the total of 14 New Jersey reactors publicly discussed, four were dropped before being officially proposed to federal regulators, six more were dropped after the proposal, and four were eventually built.

Of the four completed reactors, three are located at Salem in the southwest part of the state, and are known as Salem 1, Salem 2, and Hope Creek. The other one is Oyster Creek, located on a bay just off the Atlantic Ocean in Ocean County, in east-central New Jersey. The Salem/Hope Creek reactors were started in 1976, 1980, and 1986, while Oyster Creek began operating in 1969, making it the oldest nuclear reactor in the U.S. Each of the three Salem/Hope Creek reactors has nearly double the capacity of Oyster Creek. Combined, the reactors supply about half of New Jersey's electricity.

For years, pollution has been a public issue in New Jersey. Because the state is flanked by New York City and Philadelphia, large industrial areas on each side of the state grew during the 20th century, contaminating the state's air and water. The corridor of the northern part of the state through which the New Jersey Turnpike passes was home to many smokestack industries for years, a scenario that associated the term "New Jersey" with "polluted." The state's lengthy coastline, home to an increasing number of residents, has also been affected by various industries. The state's total of 611 Superfund sites is exceeded only by California's 781.

While nuclear reactors may not have had as high a profile as other polluters in New Jersey – such as the smokestack industries along the Turnpike or the docks of cities across from New York – they have certainly been a source of pollution. In his book Deadly Deceit, Jay Gould posted the comparative airborne emissions of each of 72 U.S. nuclear plants from 1970-1987. Oyster Creek emitted the 2nd highest amount of Iodine-131 and Particulates, which are radioactive chemicals that have a half life of over 8 days, and are most likely to enter the food chain. It also ranked 4th highest in Total Fission and Activation Gases which included those chemicals that decay very quickly.

Iodine-131 and Particulates (curies)		Fission + Activation Gases (000 curies)	
1. Dresden (IL)	95.58	1. Three Mile Island (PA)	10066
2. Oyster Creek (NJ)	**76.80**	2. Dresden (IL)	9255
3. Millstone (CT)	32.64	3. Millstone (CT)	6762
4. Quad Cities (IL)	26.79	**4. Oyster Creek (NJ)**	**5374**
5. Indian Point (NY)	17.46	5. Nine Mile Point (NY)	3698

In recent years, both Oyster Creek and Salem/Hope Creek are among the nuclear plants with the greatest environmental releases. From 2001-2004, they emitted the greatest amount of Iodine-131 in gaseous form of any U.S. nuclear plant, with the exception of LaSalle in Illinois. Radioactive iodine attacks the thyroid gland, and the large emissions from the two plants may be one reason that New Jersey's thyroid cancer rate is so high.

Oyster Creek was closed frequently for mechanical repairs. In its first 25 years of operation, the reactor only operated 67% of the time. But in recent years, the rate has moved past 90%, which is good news from a revenue standpoint, but worrisome news from a health standpoint. An aging reactor with increasingly brittle parts being run more of the time might raise the chance of a major accident, along with levels of routine radioactive emissions.

Every year, over 45,000 New Jersey residents are diagnosed with cancer. Only recently has a national cancer incidence data base been made public, with 43 states plus the District of Columbia. For the period 2000-2002, New Jersey was #1 - the highest cancer incidence rate of any state in the nation. (Its cancer death rate was 21st, suggesting that the state's relatively affluent residents could afford more life-saving cancer treatments).

Incidence rates for some cancers most affected by radiation exposure are generally high in New Jersey. The childhood cancer (age 0-19) rate is 8th highest, as over 400 children in the state are diagnosed with the disease each year. The rate of thyroid cancer, which is highly susceptible to radioactive iodine, is 2nd highest, trailing only the neighboring state of Pennsylvania.

Other cancers are affected by bone-seeking radioactive chemicals – including Strontium-90 -- that penetrate into the bone marrow and damage blood forming organs. Again, the 2000-2002 incidence rate in New Jersey is higher than most states:

Type of Cancer	New Jersey Rank In Cancer Rate, 2000-02
- All Cancers Combined	# 1
- Thyroid Cancer	# 2
- Multiple Myeloma	# 3
- Non-Hodgkin's Lymphoma	# 3
- Bone and Joint Cancer	# 4
- Hodgkin's Disease	# 6
- Leukemia	#13

With such a large penetration of nuclear reactors, and with such a high rate of cancer, especially those most susceptible to radiation exposure, it was inevitable that health concerns of nuclear reactors would become a public issue in New Jersey. While the same issues of health and safety hold for both plants, it was Oyster Creek that took most of the headlines. Perhaps it was the larger number of people living near Oyster Creek. Ocean and Monmouth Counties lie to the north of the reactor, within 40 miles. The stiff ocean breezes originating mainly from the south put these two counties in the downwind direction. Many are making a new home in the area, mostly in seashore towns; currently there are about 1.2 million residents in the two counties, nearly triple the 1960 figure. Salem County, on the other hand, is largely a rural county, with a population of only about 65,000. The facts that the shore attracts millions of visitors each summer, and counts many additional part-time residents also raise the number of those vulnerable to Oyster Creek.

Another reason that Oyster Creek came into focus for health and safety reasons is its status as the oldest reactor in the U.S. On May 3, 1969, when the reactor first produced radioactive chemicals, there were 19 nuclear power reactors operating in the U.S. All had closed by 1997, and in 2004 Oyster Creek broke the record for longest-operating reactor in U.S. history. The reactors at Salem/Hope Creek, on the other hand, are much newer; Hope Creek is actually the 18th newest of the 104 U.S. reactors.

High cancer rates near Oyster Creek were first officially measured by the National Cancer Institute in its 1990 study of cancer deaths near nuclear reactors. From the late 1960s (before Oyster Creek startup) to the 1970s and early 1980s (after startup), there was a rise in cancer deaths in Ocean

County relative to the nation. For example,

- Child cancer deaths (<20) went from 25% below the U.S. rate to 13% below
- cancer deaths for all ages went from 4% above to 10% above
- leukemia deaths went from 13% below to 1% below
- female breast cancer deaths went from equal to the U.S. to 12% higher

But these figures languished in the voluminous NCI books, and received no local attention. A check of official mortality data showed that in the two decades after 1984 the cancer death rate under age 20 had jumped to 5% ABOVE the national rate, ending years of low rates. Death rates for all cancers, leukemia, and breast cancer stayed above the U.S. Thus, Ocean County's status as a low-cancer area had been replaced by a high cancer area.

The small size of Oyster Creek, compared to Salem/Hope Creek, makes it much less of a viable economic factor, perhaps reducing any resistance to public airing of public health concerns from government and industry. Oyster Creek has a capacity of 619 Megawatts electrical, 11th lowest of the 104 U.S. reactors. The three reactors at Salem/Hope Creek have a combined capacity of 3243, second only to the Palo Verde plant in Arizona as the largest in the country. In the 1990s GPU Nuclear Corporation wanted to rid itself of the small reactor that frequently closed down, but found no buyers. In 1998, GPU announced that it was shutting the plant. But just two years later, the plant was sold, to two much larger utilities outside the state, which kept Oyster Creek running.

As ownership of Oyster Creek was being juggled, a public health uproar took place right in the reactor's back yard. In March 1996, the Newark Star-Ledger obtained data from the New Jersey Cancer Registry, and published results in a page-one headline. Rates of cancer in children who lived in Toms River NJ were exceptionally high, especially brain cancer. The next year, federal and state health officials declared an official cancer cluster, something which is rarely done.

Citizens spoke out publicly, expressing outrage at the fact that the information had not been made public by the health department. "Five weeks ago, when the report came out in the Newark Star Ledger, was the first time we heard there was a problem," said Toms River Mayor Bud Aldrich. Public pressure for answers were met by blank responses, as related by local pediatrician Julian Auerbach:

> "During a visit parents bring it up: 'What is going on? Should we drink the water? Is something causing cancer?' And we just don't know. We have absolutely no information."

The public expression of outrage was especially strong from those who had a child victimized by cancer. Local resident Linda Gillick, whose son Michael was diagnosed with neuroblastoma as a baby, organized a group Citizens Action Committee on Childhood Cancer Cluster, to oversee the investigation of the cluster, and another called Oceans of Love, a support group for the families.

The Toms River case was given a touch of star quality when Jan Schlichtmann became interested. Schlichtmann was an attorney who became famous when the book and movie A Civil Action chronicled his efforts to win a case in Woburn Massachusetts on behalf of children with leukemia who lived near toxic chemicals. He heard about the Toms River situation and began helping Gillick and the other local families with a legal action against Ciba Geigy and Union Carbide, two polluting industries with locations in the Toms River area. Schlichtmann also conferred with Gould about the tooth study, as his failure to win the Woburn case was due partly to identify contamination levels in sick children's bodies.

Along with Ciba-Geigy and Union Carbide, the possibility that radiation from Oyster Creek had harmed young children was raised. Dr. Helen Caldicott, who founded the anti-nuclear Physicians for Social Responsibility, visited Toms River in June 1996 and declared that Oyster Creek should be considered a potential contributor to the child cancer cluster.

The extensive media coverage of the cluster forced the government to take action. Just after the official cluster was declared, federal and state health officials began a review on environmental causes of the cluster. After nearly six years the $10 million study was released in December 2001. The government found a potential link between leukemia in girls diagnosed before age five if their mother had drank contaminated water while pregnant – but found no other links other than this narrow one. Even then, cautioned state epidemiologist Dr. Eddy Bresnitz "chance cannot be excluded as a possible explanation for the findings."

As for Oyster Creek, the report found no link between the reactor's emissions and the childhood cancer cluster. It made the point that actual emissions were far less than the federally-permitted levels, and estimated that emissions would cause one extra cancer death for every BILLION people – essentially stating it was harmless. Although the report ended the official study of the cluster, many were disappointed with the lack of answers explaining why so many children developed cancer.

Because health officials were highly unlikely to find any link between polluters and the cancer cluster, the door was wide open for the public and independent scientists to make their own attempt. Because of the public uproar over the child cancer cluster in Toms River, RPHP chose the area as a focus for the Tooth Fairy Project. In early 1999, it mailed several thousand letters signed by Alec Baldwin to local families appealing for donations of baby teeth. Baldwin, a Long Islander who had no special ties to New Jersey, was very moved by the child cancer situation in Toms River, and made it his focus. Over a 12 month period from early 1999 to early 2000, he made four trips to the region, each to make a public presentation on behalf of the tooth study. On one occasion, Christie Brinkley joined him on the panel.

Baldwin's visits drew considerable attendance and press attention. On November 10, 1999, over 400 people saw his presentation at Richard Stockton College in Atlantic City, where he said

> "The reason I'm here is that we have a burgeoning movement. We want to get answers about low-level radiation and exposure to it."

At the same time the tooth study took off in New Jersey, local residents organized to oppose Oyster Creek, calling the group Jersey Shore Nuclear Watch. The group was headed by Edith Gbur, a retired social worker who had moved to the area with her husband in the early 1990s. Gbur recalls that she became involved after hearing Baldwin speak at the local community college in 1999. Jersey Shore quickly became a partner of the Tooth Fairy Project. Gbur explains:

> "We thought the tooth study was very important because of the cancer situation here, especially the Toms River cancer cluster. Whether or not there's an accident or act of sabotage, the cancer

issue is the most immediate."

Local retiree Barbara Bailine became a prominent force in collecting baby teeth. Bailine, concerned about the health threat of Oyster Creek, had joined Jersey Shore Nuclear Watch, and became interested in the baby tooth study. She had RPHP send her tooth envelopes and flyers and began handing them out at public places. But at first, people paid little attention to her. Bailine began to think about how to attract attention.

> "I decided to dress up as the tooth fairy. I jazzed it up as much as I could, and made a costume by finding clothes in various stores, and sewing them into a costume."

Bailine was right – people now began to talk to the "Tooth Fairy." She went to the local mall various times with her sister, and set up a small booth with baby tooth information. "It was the mothers of small children who were most interested," she recalls. Bailine also went to parades, the local community college, the local PTA, and even made a presentation to a dental hygienist meeting. Her efforts drew considerable attention from the media, and New Jersey teeth began flowing in to RPHP.

Gbur left flyers at various locations, including stores, dentist's offices, the local mall, and the state teacher's union meeting in Atlantic City. "We had especially good luck in day care centers," she explained. The group's web site featured information on the study, and in 2001, it placed a billboard message on a local highway stating "Childhood Cancer Goes Down When Nuclear Plants Shut Down" citing the work of Mangano and RPHP.

The work was so successful that government leaders were approached for support. In 2000, a local state senator and assemblyman were instrumental in getting a measure passed calling for $75,000 in state aid for the tooth study. But Governor Christine Todd Whitman used a line-item veto to block the aid, stating that RPHP "should apply for a grant or explore private or federal funding." Baldwin shot back at Whitman's decision:

> "I am disappointed that Governor Whitman would veto such a modest appropriation that would have done so much to investigate the impacts of the Oyster Creek reactor upon local health. Clearly, public health and objective analysis are not Governor Whitman's priorities."

Three years later, RPHP made another attempt for state funding. With hundreds of New Jersey baby teeth already collected, the focus was on teeth from children with cancer. If enough baby teeth were collected from children with cancer, their Sr-90 levels could be compared with healthy children. In health research, this was called a "case-control study", in which children with cancer would be the cases and healthy children the controls.

This time, RPHP was taking no chances, and chose to deal with politicians without any public fanfare. "Under the radar screen was the way to go," says Mangano. "The industry couldn't sway any politicians if they didn't know what was going on." With the blessing of the Democratic leadership in Trenton, a two-line item calling for $25,000 for RPHP to collect and test baby teeth from children with cancer was inserted in the monstrous 300 page budget bill. On the night of June 30, 2003, just hours before the state ran out of funds, the legislature passed the budget package, with the RPHP provision virtually unnoticed.

Group members braced for another battle with the health department, which was responsible for doling out the money. Having just gone through a long battle in Westchester, nothing was certain. Four months after the budget had passed, no funds had been sent to RPHP. But a new ally of the group changed that. Earlier that year, Mangano had contacted Deirdre Imus at Hackensack University Medical Center in northern New Jersey. Deirdre was passionate about health and wellness. She was also the wife of radio personality Don Imus, who had long been involved in the Tomorrow Children's Fund, which helped children with cancer. She had begun the Deirdre Imus Environmental Center for Pediatric Oncology at Hackensack. Much of her work had been in helping children with cancer, such as the camp she and her husband ran each summer in New Mexico. But Deirdre was also interested in cancer prevention, and especially in environmental causes. The Center's Mission Statement says:

> "Nine in ten cancers can be directly traced to environmental factors: the air we breathe, the food we eat, our exposure to lead, pesticides, tobacco products, automotive and industrial emissions, even the water we drink. Regrettably, it is children who are the most vulnerable to many environmental insults."

As one way to reduce cancer through removing environmental contamination, Deirdre had begun a crusade a hospital "greening the cleaning" program, encouraging hospitals to use cleaning products with no harmful chemicals.

In mid-2003, at the suggestion of RPHP advisor (and mother of a son with leukemia) Agnes Reynolds, Mangano contacted Deirdre Imus. After a phone call and meeting, she was quite taken with the tooth study, and volunteered her help. After Mangano gave a presentation at Hackensack, Deirdre offered to hold a press conference at the hospital to kick off the effort to collect teeth from children with cancer. She lined up heavyweights such as hospital CEO John Ferguson and pediatric cancer director Michael Harris as speakers. Cory Furst, the boy with the remarkable story of overcoming lung and liver cancer, also agreed. And just hours after Deirdre appeared on her husband's show to make an appeal for New Jersey Governor James McGreevey to attend, McGreevey's office phoned in with his commitment to speak.

The November 12 event was well attended and covered. Cory Furst gave a poised appeal for tooth donations ("I'm asking all children out there who have had cancer to donate their teeth to a participating hospital."). Governor McGreevey spoke warmly of the project ("What we do here today…is take another step forward in investigating the causes of cancer.") But perhaps the most powerful words came from Dr. Harris, who reiterated the ultimate health care goal – prevention.

> "It is my fervent hope one day that we will be able to close the Tomorrow Children's Institute because we will have found what causes childhood cancer and therefore no longer will any child have to suffer the ravages of this disease."

Deirdre sent letters asking for tooth donations to all children with cancer in the Tomorrow Children's Fund. Nearly 50 children responded by sending a tooth, which was the largest number of "cancer teeth" ever sent to RPHP. Parents wrote on each envelope what type of cancer the child was suffering from, and when it was first diagnosed.

The final boost to RPHP that day came from McGreevey, who asked if state funds had been released yet. When Mangano told him and his aides "no" they carried word back to Trenton, and the following day the health department contacted Mangano and began the process of sending the checks.

In all, over 600 New Jersey children sent teeth to RPHP. Of these, only about 500 were counted as "New Jersey;" the others were children living in another state (mainly New York) at birth, and counted as part of that other state, since virtually all Sr-90 was taken up during and just after pregnancy. The results were best illustrated in the 293 teeth using the more sophisticated Perkin-Elmer counter. There was a sharp and steady decline in average Sr-90 until the 1980s – when there was a sudden turnaround. New Jersey children born in the late 1990s had a 55% higher average Sr-90 concentration than those born in the late 1980s. The large majority of the teeth were from Ocean and Monmouth County children.

By that time, above-ground bomb testing had stopped for three decades. Nuclear weapons reactors had stopped making bombs in the late 1980s, as the Cold War ended. Research reactors, which were small to begin with, were closing. And Chernobyl fallout was decaying. There was only one source of Sr-90 that was actually expanding during that time – nuclear power plants. Oyster Creek was aging, and operating a much larger portion of the time, as were other reactors in New Jersey, New York, and Pennsylvania. The study had identified what it couldn't have expected before it started. The table below shows the state trend, in average picocuries of Sr-90 in teeth per gram of calcium

Falling
Birth Yr.	NJ Avg. Sr-90
Bef. 1974	8.37 (9)
1974-77	6.99 (12)
1978-81	4.70 (12)
1982-85	2.90 (20)

Rising
Birth Yr.	NJ Avg. Sr-90
1986-89	2.91 (72)
1990-93	3.74 (115)
1994-97	4.51 (53)

There were some other results in New Jersey that went directly to the most pressing question, i.e. was Sr-90 linked with cancer risk? The greatest amount of information addressing this was compiled in New Jersey, and is discussed in the next chapter.

Getting results out to the public became the biggest task for RPHP. The group held three press conferences (2001, 2003, and 2006), each in the state capital in Trenton, to explain study findings. Each was covered extensively by media in New Jersey, New York City, and Philadelphia. Baldwin was at the 2003 event, and Dr. Donald Louria, a professor at the New Jersey Medical School attended the last one.

An unexpected opportunity to inform the public came in February 2005, when RPHP was invited to present findings to the New Jersey Commission on Radiation Protection. The Commission, which advises the state's governor, believed that low dose radiation exposure was not harmful to humans. Its Chair, Dr. Julie Timins, had written articles claiming that pelvic X-rays to pregnant women did not cause cancer in the fetus, a contradiction of many studies beginning in 1956 with the work of Dr. Alice Stewart. And in late 2003, Timins had written Governor McGreevey recommending that the state not give more funds to RPHP since the tooth study "has several faulty premises and hypotheses."

The Commission invited Gbur to testify, and when she asked if Mangano could also attend, she was surprised to hear a "yes" answer. Mangano testified, as did Gbur, Cory Furst and his mother Jane. Numerous members of the press were there to record the proceedings. Mangano asked the Commission to join RPHP and others in the search to identify causes of childhood cancer. He quoted a 1987 editorial in the New England Journal of Medicine that gave strong support for the idea that low-dose radiation causes cancer:

> "Low dose benzene and lead... confirm the suspicion that very low levels of toxins are capable of causing serious health effects. Perhaps it is time to reexamine whether scientific standards of proof of causality – and waiting for the bodies to fall – ought not give way to more preventive public health policies that are satisfied by more realistic conventions that lead to action sooner."

Commission members had typically operated in relative privacy, but with the cameras trained on them, they tried to sound conciliatory. "In order to determine whether these elevated Strontium levels are significant you would have to have something to contrast it with" was the statement offered by Timins – a vague statement that said nothing about the rising levels of Sr-90 in New Jersey. The Commission promised to consider the tooth study further – but the following January, produced a scathing 50 page report for the new governor, recommending that RPHP receive no further state funding.

Tooth study results in New Jersey were now positioned for perhaps the ultimate battle – the fight to keep Oyster Creek running vs. closing it. The federal government gives utility companies a 40 year license to operate a reactor, and can extend the license for 20 additional years. In the late 1990s, with many aging reactors reaching the end of their license period, utilities began asking for 20 year extensions.

The first application for license extension was granted in the spring of 2000. By the end of 2007, the Nuclear Regulatory Commission had reviewed renewal applications for 47 of the 104 U.S. reactors – and had approved 47 of 47. Utilities have either applied for or announced their intention to extend licenses for several dozen more reactors.

Nobody is certain whether reactors will run for 60 years total – or even how many will still be around when their original 40 year license expires. Because Oyster Creek will be 40 years old quite soon (spring 2009), the reactors owners considered their options for a long time. The decision to close the reactor in the late 1990s had been replaced by a wait-and-see attitude. Revenues from electricity produced reached an all time high, due to higher prices and the fact that since 2001, Oyster Creek operated a record 96% of the time.

Because the license extension process takes 4-5 years, a decision was needed by 2004 – exactly when AmerGen announced its decision to pursue 20 additional years. The oldest American nuclear reactor was going to try to extend its record. The plan drew a number of critical responses, including some from New Jersey officials. Governor McGreevey opposed the extension, calling it "an unknown and unnecessary risk to New Jersey communities." McGreevey's successor Jon Corzine also publicly opposed it "just because there's been too much concern about breakdowns. We have to be safe first and intellectually honest."

The license extension application was officially made in July 2005. The Nuclear Regulatory Commission, as mandated by law, prepared a report on environmental impacts posed by keeping Oyster Creek going for another 20 years. The report concluded that only minimal risks were involved, and did not mention actual emissions or cancer rates near the plant. RPHP testified at July 2006 and May 2007 hearings about the high levels of emissions and childhood cancer nearby, but to no avail. As of late 2007, the application was still in progress, as state officials and anti-nuclear groups continued to oppose it. The state Department of Environmental Protection filed an official motion with the federal government in 2006 trying to block the re-licensing, the first time a state agency had ever taken such an action. A coalition of New Jersey citizen groups also filed a motion to block the re-licensing effort.

CHAPTER 11
THE TOOTH FAIRY PROJECT EVOKES STRONG REACTIONS

The RPHP Tooth Fairy Project was a full story, as a research project, as a public health effort, and as a grassroots movement. But the reaction to the project was a story in itself. Although opinions spanned a spectrum from highly supportive to highly negative, it seemed that most reactions were strong ones.

The media played a key role in the tooth study. Since this was truly a "citizen-science" effort, and a national one (unlike St. Louis, which was mostly local), and because it was being run by a small group, the media was a key tool in informing Americans. And because this study took place in the "information age" the increasingly varied media available to RPHP presented opportunities.

From the outset, RPHP made a commitment to seek out the press. Beginning the study on Long Island, where the STAR Foundation was in high gear, made access to media easier. An appearance by Alec Baldwin or Christie Brinkley would increase the turnout of reporters. In addition, reporters were well aware of cancer concerns on Long Island by the time the tooth study began, due to the great uproar over breast cancer.

The media response on Long Island was indicative of how the media would cover RPHP. The local coverage was excellent. The Southampton Press, the closest paper to Jay Gould's summer home, faithfully reported on RPHP activities. Gould also used this and other papers to publish long letters about topics such as the Brookhaven Lab and breast cancer on Long Island. These letters were a good way to inform the public about radiation health issues.

But Long Island also established a pattern of national media refusing to cover the group. Brookhaven is only 60 miles from New York City, where the New York Times is located. Although it is a New York-based paper, the scope of the Times is much broader. It has the third greatest circulation among U.S. dailies, trailing just USA Today and the Wall Street Journal, so coverage from the Times is very desirable. Brookhaven was well covered by the Times, but it wouldn't touch RPHP. Until 2003, the Times coverage of the group was restricted to two small pieces in the metropolitan section.

In 2003, Times photographer Nancy Siesel attended the New York premiere of a new documentary called "Fatal Fallout" on the hazards of nuclear power and the struggle to find the truth about these risks. The documentary was by Gary Null, a nutritionist and environmentalist who had become very interested in RPHP's work, and included Gould, Sternglass, and Mangano. Siesel heard Mangano speak before the film; she later spoke with him and the two exchanged phone numbers. It turned out that the two lived just blocks away in the same Brooklyn neighborhood.

Siesel asked if the paper had ever covered the group's activities, especially the baby tooth study, and Mangano explained that RPHP was unofficially excluded by the Times. Articles by the science writers on radiation health always toed the government party line that low-dose radiation is not harmful. Siesel had an idea. If the science section was a dead end, why not try a human-interest story? Because Mangano worked out of his home office in Brooklyn, it could be done in the metropolitan section. Siesel successfully pitched the idea to her editor. On November 11, 2003 a long story, complete with photos, hit the Times. The writer was very impressed with the baby teeth kept by Mangano in the office – McDonnell kept the others – and began the story accordingly:

> "Joseph J. Mangano does not even notice the smell anymore. It hits you the moment you walk into his tiny, tidy apartment in Park Slope, Brooklyn, something musty and a little acrid, though not entirely unpleasant."

Although the article quoted numerous opponents of RPHP, it also gave a solid report on the group's mission and findings. The story no doubt startled the science writers at the Times, who knew nothing about it until publication. By flying under the radar screen, RPHP had successfully achieved widespread coverage. Other stories appeared in the USA Today (twice), the BBC, CNN, and National Public Radio.

Over time, the media coverage of RPHP was very impressive. The group held 22 press conferences from 1999-2006, where 4-5 media typically showed up. At least one television reporter was almost always present, along there with a cameraman – guaranteeing good coverage, since television reaches the most people.

Influencing media coverage was the scientific community, which had few members who would speak publicly in support of RPHP work. This reticence was affected much more by political considerations than scientific ones and had deep historical roots. Any scientist who supported the idea that low dose radiation exposure was harmful was fair game. The powerful backlash against Dr. Alice Stewart beginning in the mid-1950s after discovering that prenatal X-rays raised risk of childhood cancer was the first example.

Things in the U.S. got ugly as well. Dr. John Gofman of Lawrence Livermore Laboratory in California lost his large federal grant after concluding that above-ground bomb testing had caused the death of 4,000 U.S. infants. After Dr. Thomas Mancuso concluded that workers at the Hanford nuclear weapons plant suffered from high rates from cancer, the U.S. Energy Department had terminated him, with the official pronouncement that he had reached "retirement age." (Dr. Mancuso was 64 and healthy at the time, and would live until age 92). Sternglass was subject to much criticism as well, surviving professionally only because he held a tenured faculty position.

With this legacy of suppression as a backdrop, the comments from scientists came down hard on RPHP. At first, few actually commented, but especially after results of the tooth study began to get attention, the adjectives began flying. Dr. Gilbert Ross, a physician from the industry-funded American Council of Science and Health, was among the more blunt critics:

> "This report that I have read is, from an epidemiological point of view, a piece of garbage. It is a polemic, designed to attack nuclear power as an energy source."

> "The study is alarmist hyperbole of the worst sort. The risk of adverse health effects from strontium-90, whatever the source, is extremely remote bordering on zero."

Dr. Stephen Musolino, a physicist at Brookhaven Laboratories, was just as negative and dismissive, and used the common epithet of "junk science":

> "This study is ice cream science. There are more drownings in the summer. Therefore ice cream causes drowning. I'm opposed to this study because it is junk science."

The critics consistently claimed that the RPHP tooth study was not reputable, and would not stand up to the scrutiny of experts – deliberately ignoring the five medical journals that eventually published articles on the tooth study.

Mangano frequently reminded reporters that criticism of RPHP is also criticism of the many expert reviewers for journals who accepted RPHP work for publication. Critics also gave no evidence of what the "correct" levels of Strontium-90 in baby teeth should be near nuclear plants – since no other study similar to RPHPs had been done. They insisted repeatedly that any Sr-90 in baby teeth had to be left over from bomb test fallout prior to 1963 – but gave no explanation for this conclusion, other than bomb fallout levels were much greater than nuclear reactor emissions.

One frequent opponent of the tooth study was Dr. Letty Lutzker, a radiologist who lived in Westchester County NY and worked in New Jersey – both target areas for the tooth study. On two occasions, Lutzker published letters in local newspapers on the very morning that RPHP was planning a press conference on the tooth study – an indication that she and perhaps others were monitoring RPHP. Lutzker didn't just state her opposition to the tooth study, she distorted and ignored facts. In a 2003 interview to a New Jersey paper, she claimed that "reams" of studies showed no increase in cancer after nuclear plants opened – even though the 1990 National Cancer Institute study was the only such examination of the topic:

> "In a word, yes, its junk science. Miniscule strontium is emitted by nuclear plants. We have studies by reputable organizations and institutes that don't show any increase in cancer related to nuclear plants…reams of studies around nuclear plants showing no increase in cancer in any age group before and after the plants open."

However, there were some scientists who spoke out in the face of the criticism – and in defiance of government and industry – to support RPHP. Dr. Samuel Epstein, a public health professor at the University of Illinois at Chicago, was interviewed for the 2003 New York Times article and stated about RPHP "I think they are producing solid scientific work that stands critical peer review." A large boost for the tooth study came in 1999, when RPHP publicly released the initial results, based on about 500 teeth tested. Experts were needed to state their support, and RPHP went for one of the most distinguished. Dr. Victor Sidel was a professor at the Albert Einstein College of Medicine in New York City, who had been past president of the American Public Health Association. Sidel was joined by Dr. Jack Geiger, also a New York City professor who had been president of the public health group. Both were impressed with the study and gave this statement, which RPHP used more than once:

"If the levels of Strontium-90 in children's teeth and the variations in level by geographic area reported in this study are validated by appropriate repetition, these findings would appear to justify intensive follow-up and continuing large-scale surveillance. Given the biological risk associated with body burdens of even small amounts of long-lived radioactive Strontium-90, it would be prudent to regard these findings as suggestive of a potential threat to human health."

Dr. Donald Louria was also one of RPHPs supporters. Louria was a professor of preventive medicine at the New Jersey Medical School in Newark, who inserted himself early on into the battle over the troubled Oyster Creek reactor. In 2005, Louria wrote an op-ed in a New Jersey newspaper, speaking out against the dangers posed by keeping Oyster Creek going, and partly crediting RPHP and its tooth study with developing the evidence for this danger:

"Studies such as those of Joseph Mangano, national coordinator for the Radiation and Public Health Project, and colleagues measuring body burdens of that dangerous radioactive isotope, strontium, and relating those body burdens to cancer risk are very useful and important."

Louria also spoke at the March 2006 press conference at the state capitol in Trenton announcing the RPHP article linking Sr-90 in baby teeth with risk of childhood cancer near nuclear plants in New Jersey and New York. He praised the study, and challenged federal regulators to take responsibility for conducting similar studies instead of leaving it to small groups such as RPHP. "The findings make it clear that government officials must consider health risks when making nuclear policy decisions and that independent researchers should not be the only ones examining in-body radiation levels near U.S. nuclear plants" said Louria.

One of the best assessments of the hoopla caused by the RPHP tooth study was made by Stephen Lester, science director of the Commission for Health and Environmental Justice, when he said "This touches a nerve in the nuclear power industry. These plants are releasing small quantities of low-level radiation every day. The amount may seem insignificant, but when you look at 50 cities, you can see it slowly has an impact."

Another party with a major interest in the RPHP tooth study was health departments. For years, health officials at the federal level had ignored the issue of whether radioactive releases from nuclear plants raised risk of cancer for people near the plant. The 1990 study by the National Cancer Institute was just a one-time effort, only because Senator Edward Kennedy had mandated it. The Washington health establishment had left reactors to the Nuclear Regulatory Commission – which employed no health professionals, but mostly people who had worked for nuclear plants, and was funded largely by industry.

While federal health officials stayed away from the tooth study, state and local health departments jumped right in. There was no mandate for state health departments to do studies of cancer near reactors, and they like federal officials they made no comment on radiation risk near reactors – until RPHP began testing teeth. Their position was consistent regardless of the state or the reactor – that reactors emitted too little radiation to harm people, even children.

In Florida, the great public concern over the child cancer epidemic in Port St. Lucie and the RPHP tooth study near the St. Lucie plant moved David Johnson, the Florida Health Department's Chief of Environmental Epidemiology, Florida Health Department to blast the RPHP tooth study, even claiming (in the face of solid facts to the contrary) that local child cancer rates were not elevated.

> "RPHP has implied that there are large increases in cancer rates and they attribute these increases to radiation exposure from Turkey Point and St. Lucie power plants. Using this data, we have not identified any unusually high rates of cancer in these counties.
>
> There is no quantifiable risk associated with these small traces of Sr-90 in the body, even in infants. Virtually all of the environmental Sr-90 is from past nuclear weapons tests rather than power reactors, and no member of the public is receiving more than a trivially small radiation dose of any kind from the operation of nuclear power plants in the U.S."

In some areas, health departments were dispatched to keep funds out of RPHP hands. On Long Island, the Suffolk County legislature appropriated $35,000 for the tooth study in 2000. But the county executive, pressured by the nuclear industry, was determined that RPHP would not get a cent. John Matuszek, a retired state health department radiation official, was hired by the county to evaluate the tooth study, and found a host of what he termed "scientific flaws," even though he had never been involved in testing radiation in bodies. With the seal of approval from a health "expert" the county executive held up the money for nine months, and announced that no laboratory could meet the county's standards for a tooth study. The $35,000 was never released.

Another dogfight for RPHP money where health officials were called in to do the dirty work took place the following year in Westchester County NY. Again, the county legislature had appropriated funds to support the tooth study, this time $25,000. The matter was turned over to the county health department – which was taking orders from the county executive, who in turn was being leaned on by the nuclear industry.

The health department's assistant commissioner wrote Mangano a letter asking questions about the study. The letter was promptly answered – only to be followed by a second letter, asking different questions. When the number of such letters reached four, Mangano realized that the health department was stalling, and went to the press. The July 6, 2001 issue of the Westchester Weekly printed a story entitled "Cutting Their Teeth: The Radiation and Public Health Project is Still Waiting for a State Grant." Soon after the article appeared, the health department buckled and released the funds.

But the Westchester County health department wasn't through with RPHP yet. Dr. Joshua Lipsman, who directed the department, turned his full force against the group. Lipsman, who had no training or experience in the radiation health issue, commented freely to reporters and wrote letters to newspapers. "What they do is what's popularly referred to as 'junk science'" said Lipsman. "We found a number of scientific errors, both in measurement and process, in their proposals."

In August 2003, Lipsman unleashed his most vehement opposition. Mangano was holding a press conference that day at the county medical center, announcing publication of an article in the Archives of Environmental Health documenting high child cancer levels near many U.S. nuclear plants, including Indian Point in Westchester County. Lipsman entered the back of the auditorium unannounced, and sat through the proceedings. At the end of the press conference, he gathered reporters around him and unleashed a tirade against RPHP. State Assemblyman Richard Brodsky, who had spoken in support of the article, quickly went up to Lipsman and the two engaged in a verbal battle in front of reporters. Brodsky started it by asking if Lipsman had read the study, which he hadn't.

Lipsman: "I'm planning to speak after reading it as well. But in advance, I think the public needs to know this is junk science."
Brodsky: "How do you know if you haven't read it?"
Lipsman: "This is a bogus group."
Brodsky: "The statistical connection has been made. What more do you need to take appropriate public health protective steps?"
Lipsman: "There's enough controversy about Indian Point in this community without generating unnecessary garbage like this."

Yet another battleground in which the health department was called upon by politicians to smother funds for RPHP was Connecticut. In late 2004, Mangano and Agnes Reynolds had made a request to Governor Jodi Rell for $25,000 to cover costs of collecting and testing baby teeth in Connecticut children – some of whom had cancer. Rell was a moderate Republican and a breast cancer survivor herself who was moved by the tooth project, and she gave the OK to move funds into the health department. The bureaucracy moved slowly, but by November 2005, the funds had been moved and all the paperwork had been completed and was only awaiting payment to RPHP. An October 17, 2005 memo from health department fiscal officer Catherine Kennelly authorized the funds – which probably meant that she didn't know that the nuclear industry was strongly against it:

> "As discussed, we agree to provide the sum of $25,000 as requested for a study analyzing the effects of in-body radiation levels associated with strontium-90 in baby teeth. The Radiation and Public Health Project (RPHP) will be able to collect and test 150 baby teeth from Connecticut…Studies such as this are important in the attempt to identify factors contributing to the rise in childhood cancer, so that preventive strategies can be developed."

But on December 12, everything changed. The anti-nuclear group Connecticut Coalition Against Millstone held a press conference at the steps of the state capitol, charging that a high reading of Strontium-90 in milk near Millstone was evidence that the reactor was harming people. Coalition leader Nancy

Burton even brought the goat that gave the milk sample, named Katie, to the capitol. Burton and her supporters demanded to be let in to meet with Governor Rell. The event got lots of media attention, and was brought to health officials, who were asked to write a rebuttal report. Officials easily made the connection between Strontium-90 in goat's milk and Strontium-90 in baby teeth. The RPHP funds were doomed. The death knell came in a terse email on March 30, 2006 from health department official Ardell Wilson to Mangano:

> "The Department of Public Health will not execute the contract with the Radiation and Public Health Project at this time. The contract is being held pending the findings of a Connecticut Department of Environmental Protection study (not yet finished) that will address much of the same issues as the Radiation and Public Health Project."

Of course, the state study did not address the issue of child cancer, but only tried to put down the high Sr-90 reading in milk.

Regulators also were not shy about commenting about the Tooth Fairy Project. The U.S. Nuclear Regulatory Commission, as the chief regulatory agent for nuclear reactors, was heard the loudest. When preparing assessments of environmental risks for nuclear plants where RPHP was active, the NRC included strong rebuttals of the tooth study – clearing the way for their typical conclusion that reactors posed no harm to the public. The NRC went further, by placing an 8-page critique of the tooth study on its web site in December 2004.

The critique stated that "NRC finds there is little or no credibility in the studies published by the Radiation and Public Health Project." Some of the issues raised by the NRC flew in the face of basic facts. It claimed RPHP used "very small samples" – even though the tooth project was the second largest such study ever. It claimed RPHP "had not established control populations for study" – when RPHP had compared differences in children who did and didn't live close to reactors.

Most amazingly, it charged RPHP "had not subjected their data to the independent peer review of the scientific community" – closing its eyes to the fact that the tooth study had been published in five journal articles, out of the RPHP total of 22. It cited studies that showed no effect on local rates near nuclear power plants from the National Cancer Institute, University of Pittsburgh, Connecticut Academy of Sciences and Engineering, American Cancer Society, Florida Bureau of Environmental Epidemiology, and the Illinois Public Health Department. Ironically, only the first two of these had their results published in medical journals, which won't publish articles until experts approve them.

But criticism more vehement than the government/NRC came from the nuclear industry. The chief mouthpiece for industry was the Nuclear Energy Institute, a powerful Washington-based lobbying group that spoke for utilities that operated reactors. NEI frequently was critical of RPHP, terming them "an anti-nuclear citizens group based in Manhattan that has a long-range goal of closing down nuclear power plants in the United States." In July 2006, NEI unleashed a 12 page attack that appeared on its web site. The Institute spared no kind word in putting down the group and the tooth study:

> "For several decades, a small group of activists has tried to instill fear in the public that a substance called strontium-90 is evidence that low levels of radiation released from nuclear power plants causes cancer and other health problems in nearby residents. Since the claims first surfaced some 30 years ago, they continuously have been dismissed by mainstream scientists as scare tactics and 'junk science' contributing nothing to finding the real causes of cancer They are instead manipulations of the public by these groups without any basis in science. These studies are known as the 'tooth fairy project'."

NEI and individual utility companies frequently compared notes about RPHP and the tooth project, using the same arguments and citing the same sources. The power of the nuclear industry cannot be underestimated. Companies like Exelon, Entergy, and Dominion not only run multi-billion dollar operations with soaring stock prices, they also spend large amounts on political campaigns – and thus, any government official that takes an opposing side invites trouble. Paul Rosengren, of PSEG Power, which runs the Salem/Hope Creek nuclear plant in New Jersey, cautioned potential opponents to the tooth study: "Anyone who wants to be associated with this study should be careful that they're not embarrassed in the long run."

Because of this pressure, political leaders have almost uniformly been pro-nuclear, or at least noncommittal about the issue. At the federal level, the NRC under both Democratic and Republican presidents has staunchly supported the development of nuclear power. A few Congressional critics of nuclear reactors have surfaced; but these have been few in number. Often, members of Congress whose seat is "safe" and do not have to face a tough re-election campaign, such as Rep. Edward Markey and Sen. Edward Kennedy, both of Massachusetts, have been the most outspoken critics.

The baby tooth study had limited penetration in Congress. Rep. Maurice Hinchey of New York, a long time opponent of the Indian Point plant, sent a supportive letter to the RPHP press conference in Westchester County in 2000. Rep. Michael Forbes of Long Island actually appeared at an RPHP press conference in Washington – but Forbes lost his seat in the election that November.

The absence of leadership at the federal level left it to local politicians to pick up the ball. In most areas where the tooth study was active, there was one elected official that made it a priority, and spoke out publicly in favor of it. Presenting results in public was the factor that garnered support. In 2001, RPHP reported that Brick, a town in New Jersey just north of the Oyster Creek plant, had the highest average Sr-90 in baby teeth in the state. The town's Mayor Joseph Scarpelli later acknowledged that the study "made me realize that Oyster Creek was a problem. The Tooth Fairy Project was the catalyst that got me involved." Two New Jersey state assemblymen, Reed Gusciora and Matthew Ahearn, spoke at a May 2003 RPHP press conference in favor of the study, and the following month, placed the request for $25,000 in state support for the tooth study into the 2003 budget bill, which was passed by the legislature and signed by the governor.

Presenting tooth results in Westchester County in November 2000 spurred county legislator Tom Abinanti to take action and submit a bill to his legislature. Abinanti remarked after hearing from RPHP members, including Alec Baldwin:

> "My own response to what I heard here this morning is that Indian Point is a time bomb slowly going off in the mouths of our children."

In Pottstown PA, where the Limerick nuclear plant was located, Mayor Ann Jones spoke at a January 2001 press conference that kicked off the tooth study in the area. Jones gave the project a boost by calling her five-year old granddaughter to the podium, where the girl handed Mangano her tooth in the tooth study envelope. Two years later, Mangano returned to announce study results, and Jones made a statement that the local area, beset with twin problems of high childhood cancer rates and high Sr-90 levels in teeth, was being threatened by Limerick:

> "It has now been confirmed that they (the children) are also at risk from Limerick's radiation. We now know that radiation gets into the bodies of our children. That our children are far more vulnerable. That there is no safe exposure. And that on average more children have cancer here than anywhere else."

Another player in the RPHP tooth study was advocacy, or anti-nuclear groups, whose reactions paralleled that of politicians. Nationally-based groups were generally supportive, but had little to say about the study. These groups included the Nuclear Information and Resource Service, Public Citizen, the Sierra Club, the Union of Concerned Scientists, Physicians for Social Responsibility, and Greenpeace.

But at the local level, enthusiasm was great. In each area near a nuclear plant where RPHP collected at least 100 teeth, an established group played an active role in promoting the study. In New York, the STAR Foundation organized press conferences and brought out celebrity speakers to back the study. In New Jersey, the Jersey Shore Nuclear Watch took the lead. In Pennsylvania, the Alliance for a Clean Environment collected all the teeth, without the benefit of a mass mailing of appeal letters signed by Baldwin. Dr. Lewis Cuthbert, who with his wife Donna ran the Alliance, described the study in terms of human lives:

> "We don't have any expendable children that we're willing to give over to those polluters and have them wind up as victims."

Members of local advocacy groups sometimes dressed up as the "Tooth Fairy" to spur tooth donations. New Jersey retiree Barbara Bailine put together a costume with clothing purchased willy-nilly through sales, and swept through Ocean County to appeal for teeth (Chapter 9). In Westchester County NY, teacher Margo Schepart made herself a costume complete with a wand, and also made appearances, often accompanied by her young daughter. She brought her guitar with her and sang songs she had composed about the tooth project. Many were amused – but many also donated teeth.

A final group that responded to the tooth study was the public at large. Put one way, the public was generally indifferent to the study. Press conferences and public forums on nuclear power issues had modest attendance. Fewer than 5,000 teeth were donated to the project, out of the millions of children who lived near nuclear plants. Citizens did not storm Capitol Hill or state capitols demanding that action be taken on the tooth study.

But the tooth study struck a nerve in most that heard about it – especially mothers of young children. Virtually all of the donated baby teeth were sent by the child's mother, rather than the father or other adult. This pattern was similar to the St. Louis tooth study of the 1960s, when mothers such as PTA members played a prominent role in tooth collection. Mothers would call RPHP with questions such as "will my child get sick from Strontium-90?" or "we want to move to a town near a nuclear plant: is this unsafe for my child?"

Mothers of children with cancer presented a special case. Most children of those who showed interest in the tooth study had been successfully treated and were recovering (parents of those who were still sick were usually too overwhelmed physically and emotionally to get involved with things like the tooth study). But after their child had recovered, the question shifted from "will my child live?" to "why did my child get cancer?" With few known factors for childhood cancer, the tooth study had an appeal to many of these curious women.

CHAPTER 12
TOOTH STUDIES - LINKS WITH CHILD CANCER AND LEGACIES

In mid-2006, the RPHP Board of Directors decided to temporarily halt the Tooth Fairy Project. The study had achieved, even exceeded, all the goals that were originally set a decade earlier. Over 4,700 baby teeth had been collected and tested, very close to Jay Gould's original target of 5,000. Results had been published in five medical journal articles. Results showed consistent and significant patterns of Strontium-90 levels in teeth. Counties closest to reactors had levels 30-50% higher than more distant counties, and average Sr-90 had increased about 35-60% since the late 1980s. These were clear indications that reactor emissions were entering children's bodies.

The most important question addressed by the study was whether these relatively-low levels of radioactivity caused cancer. This question had been posed nearly half a century ago during the period when St. Louis researchers studied Sr-90 from bomb fallout in baby teeth, and government programs examined Sr-90 in bone. Unfortunately, virtually no attempt to link this radiation with cancer risk was made. Three medical journal articles in the 1960s had compared Sr-90 concentration in bones of persons with and without cancer. The studies used small samples and were inconclusive – and not followed up for nearly 40 years.

So after decades, and after the great efforts made scientists from Washington University, RPHP, and foreign experts, have in-body studies of Strontium-90 shown that low doses of radioactivity from nuclear weapons and reactors cause cancer – especially in children?

The answer to this question is not a blanket "yes" or "no" but is actually part of a detective story in which clues and evidence are collected, step by step. So far, in 2007, here's what clues have been found.

1. _Strontium-90 Causes Cancer in Lab Animals_. For years, scientists have known that radioactive strontium caused cancer. In 1945, University of Chicago scientists began an experiment in which dogs were injected with Strontium-90. The dogs and their puppies suffered from a lack of weight gain, cancer, pneumonia, and other immune-related diseases. At death, measurements showed high levels of Sr-90 in the dogs, indicating that it stayed in the body for a long time.

2. <u>Low Doses of Radiation Cause Cancer in Children</u>. The 1950s and early 1960s were a pivotal time for better understanding the Sr-90/childhood cancer connection. The theory that low doses of radiation could cause children to develop cancer were given strong supporting evidence, first by Dr. Alice Stewart as she showed that a single pelvic X-ray to pregnant British women in the mid-1950s nearly doubled the chance that the child would die from cancer by age ten. Stewart's study was duplicated by Dr. Brian MacMahon shortly thereafter.

In the 1960s, studies were conducted on Sr-90 effects in animals. This time, only a small dose of the chemical was injected into lab rats. Even at these low doses, a decline in blood cells in the bone marrow were observed, indicating that the Sr-90 had attached to the bone and penetrated into bone marrow, where cell destruction occurred. Other experiments showed that Sr-90 lowered the number of Natural Killer cells in animals. These cells are critical in fighting cancer.

In 2005, a blue ribbon panel of the National Academy of Sciences issued a report concluding that any dose of radiation carried health risk (including cancer), based on many professional articles. Just two years earlier, the U.S. Environmental Protection Agency issued a draft paper stating that a radiation dose to children under age two carries 10 times the risk of the same dose to adults. These two official documents give further basis for the belief that small doses of Sr-90 have caused cancer in children.

3. <u>More Bomb Testing, More Sr-90, More Childhood Cancer</u>. U.S. childhood cancer rates soared during the 1950s and early 1960s, while over 200 atomic weapons were exploded above the ground in the South Pacific and Nevada, sending large clouds of radioactive fallout into the air, and later into the food chain and human bodies. And after the Partial Test Ban Treaty ended large-scale tests, in-body radioactivity levels plunged along with childhood cancer rates.

The distinct patterns of childhood cancer rising and falling with fallout levels gave researchers a chance to further examine a Sr-90/childhood cancer link. The St. Louis baby tooth study, which showed a buildup of Sr-90 in bodies during testing and a decline after the treaty, could have used results to examine this link, but did not, leaving the issue unresolved.

But there was nearly a total silence from the research community on this topic.

Even relatively basic analyses of child cancer near areas hard-hit by bomb fallout were virtually non-existent. The political pressures during the Cold War period, as the United States vied with the Soviet Union for superiority in nuclear weapons, played a strong role in this topic being ignored. A 1997 National Cancer Institute study concluding that up to 212,000 Americans (almost all adults) developed thyroid cancer from exposure to fallout is the only official admission that bomb testing caused cancer.

4. *More Reactors, More Childhood Cancer.* As late as the spring of 1967, there were only 8 nuclear power reactors operating in the U.S., each of them small models. By 1990 the number had soared to 111, most of these many times larger than the original models, in 31 of the 50 states.

At the same time that reactors were proliferating, childhood cancer deaths were declining sharply, as improved methods of detection and treatment enabled doctors to save the lives of more children. But as death rates were falling sharply, incidence rates were rising just as quickly, an increase of about 30% from the early 1970s to early 1990s. This phenomenon was consistent nationwide, and for leukemia, brain cancer, and other types of cancer. No factors were offered by the medical and public health communities to explain this unexpected trend.

Scientists and citizens alike proposed that environmental pollutants, including radioactive emissions from nuclear reactors might be one factor driving up rates of childhood cancer. A number of medical journals articles were published documenting elevated rates of child cancer near nuclear plants. A number of these focused on leukemia, known to be especially sensitive to radiation exposure. These studies were still basic, but provided more evidence supporting a linkage.

But most of these papers were from the United Kingdom and other foreign countries, with only a small handful from the U.S. (the country with one-fourth of all the nuclear reactors worldwide). Again, the strong political influence of the nuclear industry and the government stood in the way of more studies being done, and criticized any results that showed a potential connection.

5. *High Rates of Child Cancer Near Three Mile Island, Chernobyl.* There was perhaps no greater opportunity to do research on man-made radioactivity and child cancer risk than after the Three Mile Island and Chernobyl accidents.

But what happened was disappointing.

For nearly 12 years after the 1979 Three Mile Island accident, no medical journal articles examined cancer rates near the plant, for children or adults. When an article was finally published, it showed a sharp rise in cancer cases within ten miles of the plant in the first five years after the accident – including child cancer. But even with this strong evidence, the Columbia University researchers who wrote the article concluded that Three Mile Island had not caused cancer – and even suggested that the high cancer rates after the accident were due to stress.

In the case of Chernobyl, which emitted much more radioactivity than Three Mile Island, there were some breakthroughs. A number of articles showed that thyroid cancer in local children soared beginning four years after the 1986 disaster. Rises in infant leukemia were also documented. But the research largely stopped at this point, and a tie-in between radiation and childhood cancer remained elusive.

6. *Counties Near Reactors Have Highest Childhood Cancer Incidence*. Looking at statewide childhood cancer rates is not very meaningful due to the large land area; county-specific data is much more precise. As mentioned earlier, few studies have ever been done examining childhood cancer rates in counties closest to nuclear reactors. Journal articles have been published on only the Oak Ridge, Hanford, and San Onofre nuclear plants. The 1990 National Cancer Institute study mandated by Senator Edward M. Kennedy examined deaths from cancer, including children, in counties closest to nuclear plants, but concluded that the data showed no link between living near a nuclear reactor and cancer risk.

Joseph Mangano recently published two articles that examined childhood cancer rates in counties closest to nuclear reactors. One examined incidence (or cases), and the other examined mortality (deaths).

The article on incidence analyzed data from counties completely or mostly within 30 miles of 14 nuclear plants in the eastern United States. Cases diagnosed in children under age ten during 1988-1997 (3669) made the study by far the most comprehensive look at childhood cancer near U.S. reactors. The results showed that local rates exceeded the national rate near 14 of 14 plants. The total excess of 12.4% was statistically significant, and translated into 455 "excess" cases out of the total of 3669 diagnosed.

The following lists the nuclear plants included in the article, and the percent above the U.S. rate near each plant. The counties nearest to two nuclear plants in Florida, Turkey Point (just south of Miami) and St. Lucie (about 150 miles north) had the highest rates of all areas studied.

Local Incidence Rates, All Cancers Age 0-9, Compared to U.S. Rate
Counties < 30 Miles of Nuclear Plants, 1988-1997

Plant (State)	% +/- U.S. Rate (Cases)
St. Lucie FL	+45.1 (76)
Turkey Point FL	+28.2 (575)
Oyster Creek NJ	+26.5 (280)
Indian Point NY	+17.4 (253)
Brookhaven NY	+16.4 (307)
Pilgrim MA	+14.6 (120)
Susquehanna PA	+12.8 (136)
Seabrook NH	+ 8.2 (250)
Peach Bottom PA	+ 7.4 (322)
Beaver Valley PA	+ 4.0 (395)
Crystal River FL	+ 3.8 (84)
Limerick PA	+ 3.3 (488)
Millstone CT	+ 2.2 (178)
Salem/Hope Cr NJ	+ 2.2 (205)

7. *Counties Near Reactors Have Rising Childhood Cancer Mortality.* The other study published by Mangano examined cancer deaths among children age 0-9 living in counties closest to nuclear reactors. Mangano reasoned that not immediately, but several years after a plant began operating, radioactive exposures to the very young would result in higher rates of childhood cancer deaths. To test his theory, he examined local child cancer death rates (vs. the U.S.) 1-5 years and 6-10 years after a plant began operating, expecting that there would be a difference between the two periods. Only the areas near plants with a substantial population were included, to increase the chances that the number of deaths would be statistically significant.

Mangano's theory proved to be correct as he published findings in 2006. The childhood cancer death rate near 20 plants started before 1982 was 1% below the U.S. in the first five years of operation, but 18% above the U.S. during the next five years.

The same finding was reached was for the 13 plants started since 1982, with local cancer rates jumping from 8% below to 5% above the U.S. The large number of deaths involved (1898) made the findings statistically significant. Increases occurred for leukemia and all other types of childhood cancer.

8. <u>Childhood Cancer Incidence Near Reactors Tumble After Shutdown</u>. In addition to examining childhood cancer increases after reactors start, the opposite can be done, i.e. examining decreases after reactors close. The 17 U.S. reactors that have closed since 1979 create an opportunity to study this issue.

Actually, this theory has its roots in the period just after the 1963 treaty ended above-ground atomic bomb tests in the U.S. Cancer incidence in children under age five in Connecticut (the only state with an established cancer registry) plunged 25.5% from 1963-64 to 1965-71. The findings fit the theory that less fallout from bomb tests would enter children's bodies and make them less susceptible to cancer. The same theory can be applied to children living near closed reactors; after reactors close, children take in less radiation from reactors, leaving them less susceptible to cancer.

In the year 2000, Mangano announced he had found large decreases in local infant deaths immediately after nuclear reactors closed. He reasoned that if infant deaths dropped, then cancer in children should do the same. He restricted his analysis to counties less than 40 miles and east/downwind of permanently closed reactors, with the nearest operating reactor at least 70 miles distant. The last two years that the reactor operated were set as the "before" period, and the following seven years were set as the "after" period.

Mangano found a sudden drop in cancer incidence in children under age five, in 6 out of 6 areas for which data were available. The total drop was 23.9%, at a time when incidence rates were rising slightly (below). This was quite similar to the 25.5% drop found after bomb testing was halted in the 1960s.

Plant	Year Closed	% Change in Cancer Inc. 0-4
LaCrosse WI	1987	-38.6%
Rancho Seco CA	1989	-25.4%
Fort St. Vrain CO	1989	-12.0%

Big Rock Point MI	1997	-53.3%
Maine Yankee ME	1997	-29.9%
Zion IL	1998	- 7.6%
TOTAL		-23.9%

9. *<u>Childhood Cancer Clusters Near Reactors</u>*. Another source of evidence supporting the belief that emissions from nuclear reactors raise childhood cancer risk is the reported clusters of childhood cancer. These have been discussed in Chapter 7, so they will only be mentioned here:

- Perhaps the largest cluster of childhood children certified by the U.S. government occurred in Toms River NJ during the 1980s and 1990s. Toms River is nine miles from the Oyster Creek nuclear reactor, the oldest of the 104 U.S. reactors.

- Another large childhood cancer cluster took place in Port St. Lucie FL, just several miles from the two St. Lucie nuclear reactors. Many of these cases were brain and nervous system cancers.

- An unusually large number of children with rhabdomyosarcoma was documented in central Long Island, the location of the Brookhaven Nuclear Laboratories.

The evidence presented here all support the theory that low doses of Strontium-90 from atomic bombs and nuclear reactors has caused Americans to develop cancer during childhood. For many lay persons familiar with this evidence, this is enough to convince them that such a link exists. But for scientists, this conclusion requires more work. Specifically, it must be demonstrated that Sr-90 is released into the air by nuclear reactors and enters human bodies. Moreover, specific levels of Sr-90 in human bodies must be documented, and assessed for cancer risk using a variety of research tools.

This is indeed a steep hill to climb. For decades, many scientists believed that cigarette smoking increased risk of lung cancer and other diseases. But it wasn't until January 1964, with the release of a landmark report by the U.S. Surgeon General containing summaries of a large array of scientific research projects, that a general and official consensus was reached on the link. For the Sr-90/childhood cancer link, considerable work must be done to reach this consensus.

The first piece of evidence that needs to be documented is that Sr-90 from nuclear reactors is emitted into the environment by nuclear reactors. The U.S. Nuclear Regulatory Commission requires that each nuclear plant operator submit an annual report including, among other things, a measurement of airborne emissions of various radioactive chemicals. A summary of these emissions are available on the internet, at www.reirs.com/effluent/EDB, beginning with the year 2001. For about half of the reactors, the level of Sr-90 is reported as "non-detectable." But for the rest, an actual amount is given in picocuries, a measure of radioactivity. Some reactors report hundreds of times greater Sr-90 emissions than others.

The next step is to document that Sr-90 from nuclear reactors is actually entering human bodies. This was not done – until RPHP began its Tooth Fairy Project. The study measured Sr-90 in over 4,700 baby teeth, many near seven U.S. nuclear plants. Two findings made it clear that most, if not all, the Sr-90 in baby teeth represented emissions from reactors: the highest levels of Sr-90 were in counties closest to reactors, and average levels had risen sharply since the late 1980s. The tables below provide actual results from a 2003 article on the tooth study. These two discoveries, which were highly significant due to the large number of teeth tested, made it clear that most of the Sr-90 in teeth had come from a current source (reactor emissions), and was not left over fallout from 1950s atomic bomb tests or emissions from the 1986 Chernobyl accident.

Plant/ Closest Counties	Number of Baby Teeth Near Reactor	Rest of State	% Avg Sr90 is +/- Rest of State
Indian Point NY (Putnam, Rockland, Westchester)	217	317	+35.8%
Limerick PA (Berks, Chester, Montgomery)	98	32	+53.2%
Turkey Point FL (Broward, Dade, Palm Beach)	350	24	+38.6%
St. Lucie FL (Martin, St. Lucie)	97	24	+53.8%
Oyster Creek NJ (Monmouth, Ocean)	169	75	+ 8.1%
Diablo Canyon CA (San Luis Obispo, Santa Barbara)	50	88	+30.8%

	No. of Teeth by Birth Year		% Increase Avg Sr90
State	'86-89	'94-97	1986-89 vs. 1994-97
California	50	20	+50.2%
Florida	102	99	+36.3%
New Jersey	71	39	+36.5%
New York	142	104	+53.6%
Pennsylvania	32	36	+27.7%
All Other	135	48	+59.0%
TOTAL	532	346	+48.5%

Now that it is clear that Sr-90 from reactors enters bodies, the next step is to correlate these Sr-90 levels with childhood cancer patterns. The tables above show elevated levels of Sr-90 near the Indian Point, Limerick, Oyster Creek, St. Lucie, and Turkey Point plants. Earlier in the chapter, high rates of childhood cancer near these same plants were shown. Conclusion: areas with high Sr-90 levels in baby teeth also have high childhood cancer rates.

Another way to assess the Sr-90/cancer link is to examine trends. In other words, when Sr-90 increases over time, does childhood cancer also increase? This is a legitimate question in health research. Levels of smoking rose steadily during the mid-20th century, followed by a steady decline. Several decades after smoking rates began to rise, lung cancer rates increased at a similar rate – and then declined at a similar rate.

In the 2006 article, Mangano included line graphs of trends in Sr-90 and cancer incidence age 0-9 near three nuclear plants (Brookhaven, Indian Point, and Oyster Creek). In each graph the two lines looked the same, i.e. increases in Sr-90 in teeth were followed by increased in childhood cancer, and decreases were followed by decreases. Because hundreds of teeth and hundreds of cancer cases were used, results were highly significant. This is the closest correlation ever published in a medical journal of the link between cancer and chemicals produced in nuclear weapons and reactors.

Another way to examine the link is to compare Sr-90 levels in the teeth of children with cancer to levels in teeth of healthy children. This method is known as a "case-control" study, and has been used extensively in health research. Comparing persons with lung cancer and healthy persons always shows many more smokers in the group with lung cancer. In 2002, RPHP began an attempt to collect baby teeth specifically from children with cancer. It secured $50,000 in grants from a foundation in Miami and the New Jersey state legislature to underwrite the costs. Pediatric cancer units in hospitals were asked for help in collecting teeth.

In all, nearly 200 teeth from children with cancer were collected. In Florida, these teeth had much higher Sr-90 levels than did healthy children. In New Jersey, levels also were higher, but the difference was much more modest. There were problems with the "cancer teeth." About one-quarter could not be analyzed, as there was not enough intact enamel for the lab to get an accurate measurement of Sr-90. More importantly, there were simply not enough teeth to obtain a good "case control" comparison. Because of these obstacles, no medical journal article was ever published on the "cancer teeth" – although the higher levels of Sr-90 should be taken seriously.

In summary, there is considerable evidence that Sr-90 from U.S. nuclear reactors has caused childhood cancer. The evidence comes from early experiments on animals, data on childhood cancer trends, and Sr-90 measurements in over 4,700 baby teeth. It is backed by medical journals, whose experts deemed the articles worthy of publication. Many informed lay persons are already convinced that there is a connection. The approval of the scientific community has not yet been completed, but future research can build on what has already been done.

The legacy of tooth studies is still emerging, but it has been significant. From its humble beginnings, when scientist Herman Kalckar suggested an "international milk tooth census" in 1958 to measure atomic bomb fallout buildup in bodies, studies of Strontium-90 in baby teeth have created quite a history. Their impact has been felt in the fields of science, public policy, and health.

<u>Impact on Science</u>. Testing radioactivity levels in human bodies is the most effective method of understanding the effects of nuclear weapons testing and nuclear reactor operations. In-body testing is commonly used not just for radioactive substances, but for other chemicals such as lead. And in-body tests of man-made radioactivity in animals have been conducted from the time when these chemicals were created.

In what should be considered one of the most amazing scientific accomplishments of the late 20th century, Washington University in St. Louis conducted a large-scale study of Sr-90 in baby teeth from bomb fallout. The St. Louis study is accepted by all but the most radical pro-nuclear factions as sound science, despite the political fires that burned around it. The sharp and consistent rise of Sr-90 concentrations in teeth as bomb tests continued, and the equally rapid plunge after they were stopped were reported in various medical journals.

The study was so successful it inspired similar efforts in many European nations. Scientists from these countries used St. Louis as a prototype, and found exactly the same patterns as in the U.S. It also was influential in the U.S. government funding studies of Sr-90 in bone, one for adults and one for children, which also documented the same pattern as the Washington University tooth study.

Baby tooth studies did not end with the St. Louis study. In the 1990s, scientists in Germany, Greece, and the Ukraine undertook studies of Sr-90 in baby teeth after the disastrous 1986 accident at the Chernobyl nuclear plant. Each study showed a large rise in Sr-90 after the Chernobyl fallout cloud passed over Europe and entered the food chain. Also in the 1990s, a research team examined Sr-90 and plutonium-239 levels in baby teeth near a nuclear plant in England. This study was also groundbreaking, as it was the first to show that radioactivity ROUTINELY emitted from a nuclear reactor actually entered the human body.

In the past decade, the latest chapter in baby tooth studies has been written by the Radiation and Public Health Project. Study findings, which were published in five medical journal articles from 2000-2006, were unexpected. Average Sr-90 levels in baby teeth were 30-50% higher in the counties closest to reactors, and levels increased by 35-60% from the late 1980s to the late 1990s. These findings provided strong evidence that a large portion of the Sr-90 in teeth represented emissions from reactors, and not fallout from Chernobyl or bomb tests conducted decades earlier.

<u>Impact on Policy</u>. Because nuclear issues are politically charged ones, the baby tooth studies did not exist in a vacuum. The St. Louis study, plus the European ones that soon followed it, were conducted as a direct response to the ongoing nuclear weapons tests that were blanketing the globe with radioactive fallout. Naturally, officials at the highest levels of government were silent at best, or outright hostile at worst. They wanted any information that suggested tests were threatening Americans to be kept quiet. Some

opponents made the "Communist" charge at the Committee on Nuclear Information, a charge totally lacking merit.

But the study took place in spite of the opposition. Scientists at Washington University and many dedicated St. Louis citizens deserve much credit for this. In 1963, five years after the study began, a treaty banning all above-ground tests was agreed to by the U.S., Soviet Union, and Great Britain. After above-ground tests stopped, levels of Sr-90 and all other chemicals found in fallout plunged rapidly, relieving Americans of much of the burden of these harmful chemicals.

The RPHP tooth study emulated the "citizen-science" model of its St. Louis predecessor by building coalitions with concerned citizens in communities near nuclear reactors. It was successful in interesting government officials, obtaining grants from governments in Westchester County NY and the state of New Jersey, plus individual legislators from New York and Pennsylvania. RPHP and others are using study results in the debate over whether to keep aging reactors running and whether to build new reactors.

Impact on Health/Childhood Cancer. The third area, along with science and public policy, on which tooth studies have had an influence, is health. The Washington University tooth study was not originally intended to be a health study, but a measurement of Sr-90 to support an end to above-ground bomb testing. However, questions were raised by the public and citizens alike that rising Sr-90 could be a risk factor for cancer, especially in children. Barry Commoner proposed doing such a health study, but the limited technology for testing teeth at that time made such an effort impossible.

RPHP was the first to examine health risks using baby tooth study results, and it concentrated on childhood cancer, the disease mostly likely to show such a risk. The group has found a statistical link between Sr-90 in teeth and cancer diagnosed in children under age ten near three nuclear plants in New Jersey and New York. The group demonstrated that when Sr-90 levels rise near a reactor, childhood cancer rates rise several years later; and when Sr-90 levels fall, childhood cancer fall. More epidemiological study is needed, but these results are significant ones.

RPHP has also found that children with cancer have higher Sr-90 levels in their baby teeth than do healthy children, although this comparison needs to be refined before it is officially published in a medical journal.

Studies of Sr-90 in baby teeth, along with other radioactive chemicals in the body, will undoubtedly continue in the future, as long as man-made fission products are part of our earth. The future role they will play in the areas of science, health, and public policy is uncertain, dependent on political will as much as it is on technical know-how.

But as long as cancer continues to proliferate in our society, and as long as finding causes and preventing disease take a back seat to detection and treatment, public interest in studies like these will continue. Ordinary citizens, some of whom suffer from cancer or who have a child with cancer, will play a vital role in this support. It may take time, but answers and policy changes are inevitable.

REFERENCES

<u>Chapter 1</u>
Allen W. Baby Tooth Study Has New Life. St. Louis Post Dispatch, November 9, 2001.

Tooth Fairy Returns. San Francisco Chronicle, November 27, 2001.

Revival of Baby Teeth Study Denounced. The Washington Post, December 2, 2001.

Allen W. Subjects of First Study Say They are Eager for New Information. St. Louis Post Dispatch, January 6, 2002.

Correspondence by letter, Ralph Quatrano to Joseph Mangano, October 2, 2001.

Correspondence by email, Nancy Schimmel to Joseph Mangano, June 15, 2003.

Personal correspondence, Daniel Kohl to Joseph Mangano, June 20, 2001.

Correspondence by email, Daniel Kohl to Joseph Mangano, June 22, 2001.

Personal correspondence, Marcia Marks, February 15, 2007.

Email from Susan Rickfels, November 9, 2001.

Email from Kelly Persons, November 10, 2001.

Email from GACATLANTA@aol.com), Gail Cordes, November 14, 2001.

Email from rnelson@Princeton.EDU, Rob Nelson, November 10, 2001.

Email from, fucoloro@earthlink.net, Debbie (Gallina) Fucoloro, November 9, 2001.

Email from poppawalt@earthlink.net, Walter J. Kent, DDS, November 12, 2001.

Letter from Elizabeth R. Brookman, Richmond Heights MO.

Email from Don Hansel, November 11, 2001.

Email from jatr@ktis.net, JoAnn Reagan, January 2, 2002.

Email from hmcn@socket.net, Helen McNally, November 12, 2001.

Email from JKDOUEZ@aol.com, Kathleen A. (Cornish) Douez, January 4, 2002.

Email from pchotin@chotingroup.com, Phyllis Chotin, November 2001.

Email from June Masek, November 19, 2001.

Email from gschwartz@shaare-emeth.org, Gail Schwartz, November 20, 2001.

Email from annef@hydrodramatics.com, Anne Marie Fox Gunn, January 16, 2002.

Email from LCulligan@aol.com, Janet (McClurken) Culligan, January 4, 2002.

Email from cayoung@decarealty.com), Caroline Young, November 2001.

Email from TLMCVEY@aol.com, Tim McVey, December 2001.

Email from rhayden@adams-tax.com, Russ Hayden, December 2001.

Chapter 2
Reynolds A. A journey called life. Advance for Nurses 2003, 23-24, 35.

Dash J. The one-in-a-hundred miracle: a New Jersey mom refuses to surrender her baby to cancer. Family Circle, April 1, 1998, 90-92.

National Center for Health Statistics. Vital Statistics of the United States; Volume II: Mortality. Washington DC: U.S. Government Printing Office. Annual volumes beginning 1937.

Surveillance, Epidemiology, and End Results (SEER), available at www.seer.gov.

Sherman W. City's Hospitals are Bleeding Red Ink. New York Daily News, February 9, 2003.

U.S. Department of Health and Human Services. Forty-five years of Cancer Incidence in Connecticut, 1935-79. NIH Publication Number 86-2652. Washington DC: U.S. Government Printing Office, 1986.

Stewart A et al. A survey of childhood malignancies. British Medical Journal 1958(i):1495-1508.

Norris RS and Cochran TB. United States Nuclear Tests, July 1945 to 31 December 1992. Washington DC: Natural Resources Defense Council, 1994.

U.S. Nuclear Regulatory Commission, www.nrc.gov.

Chapter 3
Miller R. Under the Cloud: The Decades of Nuclear Testing. New York: The Free Press, 1986.

Ball H. Justice Downwind: America's Atomic Testing Program in the 1950s. Oxford University Press, 1988.

Duck and Cover (1951 film). Available at www.archive.org/details/DuckandC1951.

"Our Friend the Atom." In Langer M. Disney's Atomic Fleet. Available at www.awn.com/mag/issue2.1.3.pages/3.1langerdisnsey.html.

Salisbury HE. Stevenson Calls for World Pact to Curb H-Bomb. The New York Times, October 16, 1956.

U.S. Public Health Service. Radiological Health Data and Reports. Monthly volumes, 1960-1971.

Kulp et al. Strontium-90 in man. Science 1957;125(3241):219-25.

Leary WE. In 1950's, U.S. Collected Human Tissue to Monitor Atomic Tests. The New York Times, June 21, 1995.

Radioactive Rise Noted, and Harriman Scores AEC's Test Halt. The New York Times, November 2, 1956.

Shute N. On the Beach. New York: William Morrow, 1957.

Pauling L. Nobel Lecture, December 11, 1963. Available at www.geocities.com/peace.

Schweitzer A. A Declaration of Conscience, April 24, 1957. Available at www.wagingpeace.org/articles.

Chapter 4
Kalckar H. An international milk teeth radiation census. Nature 1958;4631:283-4.

Sullivan WC. Nuclear Democracy: A History of the Greater St. Louis Citizen's Committee for Nuclear Information, 1957-1967. St. Louis: Washington University, University College Occasional Papers No. 1, 1982.

St. Louis Committee for Nuclear Information, Science and Citizen. Monthly volumes, 1961-1969.

Personal correspondence, Louise Reiss, February 25, 2002, May 6, 2003.

Email from sschloeman@im.wustl.edu, Suzanne Schloeman, 11/20/01.

Email from mpn@psyc.tamu.edu, Margaret Norris PhD, psychology professor at Texas A + M University, 11/10/01.

Email from PFahrendorf@smtp.sosu.edu, Pam Fahrendorf, 11/13/01.

Email from jinx@exl.com, Normagene Jenks, 11/9/01.

Email from GOLDAVID@aol.com, Golda Mantinband Cohen, 11/9/01.

Email from AnnetAdams@aol.com, Annet Adams, 11/9/01.

Email from shieber@deas.harvard.edu, Stuart M. Shieber, 11/9/01.

Email from BBabypie@aol.com, Kathy Persons, 11/10/01.

Email from vmccarthy@SCHLEEHUBER.com, Vincent McCarthy, 11/13/01.

Email from skip@sentientworks.com, Skip Cassidy, 12/9/01.

Email from Airbante@aol.com, 12/18/01.

Reiss LZ. Strontium-90 absorption by deciduous teeth. Science 1961;134:1669-73.

Rosenthal HL. Strontium-90 content of deciduous human incisors. Science 1963;340:176-7.

Pauling L. No More War! New York: Dodd-Mead, 1958.

Chapter 5
Powers FG. Operation Overflight: The U-2 Spy Tells His Story for the First Time. New York: Holt, Rinehart, and Winston, 1970.

Swerdlow A. Women Strike for Peace: Traditional Motherhood and Radical Politics in the 1960s. Chicago: The University of Chicago Press, 1993.

Sorenson TC. Kennedy. New York: Harper Collins, 1965.

Kennedy, John F. Address to the Nation, Washington DC, July 26, 1963.

Johnson, Lyndon B. Remarks at the University of New Mexico, Albuquerque NM, October 28, 1964.

Shaughnessy D. Jimmy Fund Gets 50th Anniversary Gift: "Jimmy." Boston Globe, May 17, 1998.

Dana-Farber Cancer Institute: Who was Sidney Farber? Available at https://www.dfci.harvard.edu/abo/history/who/

Greene G. The Woman Who Knew Too Much: Alice Stewart and the Secrets of Radiation. Ann Arbor MI: University of Michigan Press, 1999.

Stewart A. et al. Malignant disease in childhood and diagnostic irradiation in utero. Lancet 1956;2:447.

MacMahon B. Prenatal X-ray exposure and childhood cancer. Journal of the National

Cancer Institute 1962;28(5):1173-91.

Sternglass E. Cancer: relation of prenatal radiation to development of the disease in childhood. Science 1963;140:1102-4.

Kennedy, John F. Remarks at Press Conference, Washington DC, August 20, 1963.

Weiss ES et al. Surgically treated thyroid disease among young people in Utah, 1948-1962. American Journal of Public Health 1967;57(10):1807-14.

Chapter 6

Personal correspondence, Harold Rosenthal, April 12, 2001, August 10, 2001, November 30, 2001.

Rosenthal HL et al. Incorporation of fall-out strontium-90 in deciduous incisors and foetal bone. Nature 1964;4945:615-6.

Sternglass E. Secret Fallout: Low-Level Radiation from Hiroshima to Three Mile Island. New York: Ballantine Books, 1972.

Commoner B. Science and Survival. New York: Viking Press, 1967.

Kolehmainer L, Rytomaa I. Strontum-90 in deciduous teeth in Finland: a followup study. Acta Odontol. Scand 1975;33(2):107-10.

Starkey WE, Fletcher W. The accumulation and retention of strontium-90 in human gteeth in England and Wales – 1959 to 1965. Archives of Oral Biology 1969;14(2):169-79.

D'Arca Simonetti A et al. Determination of strontium-90 in the deciduous teeth. Annali Stomatologica 1969;18(1):23-38.

Aarkrog A. Strontium-90 in shed deciduous teeth collected in Denmark, the Faroes, and Greenland from children born in 1950-1958. Health Physics 1968;15(2):105-114.

Rosenthal HL. Accumulation of Environmental 90Sr in Teeth of Children. Hanford Radiobiological Symposium, Richland WA, May 1969, 163-171.

U.S. Public Health Service. Radiation Health Data and Reports, monthly volumes, 1962-1971 (Sr-90 in children's bones).

Klusek CK. Strontium-90 in Human Bone in the U.S., 1982. New York: U.S. Department of Energy, Environmental Measurements Laboratory, 1984 (Sr-90 in adult bone).

Personal correspondence, Sophie Goodman, August 30, 2001, September 28, 2001, October 17, 2001.

Personal correspondence, Yvonne Logan, August 28, 2001, October 24, 2003.

Correspondence by letter from Yvonne Logan to Joseph Mangano, August 20, 2001.

Moment of Tooth. Newsweek, April 25, 1960, p. 70.

Aleksandrowicz J et al. The amount of Sr90 in the bones of people who have died of leukemias. Blood 1963;22(3):346-50.

Woodard H and Harley JH. Strontium-90 in the long bones of patients with sarcoma. Health Physics 1965;11:991-8.

Sata C and Sakka M. The quantity of strontium 90 in the bone of leukemic patients. Tohoku Journal of Experimental Medicine 1968;94:45-53.

Chapter 7

Eisenhower DD. Atoms for Peace. Speech delivered at the United Nations, New York, December 8, 1953.

Strauss L. Speech delivered to National Association of Science Writers, New York, September 16, 1954. Reported in the New York Times, September 17, 1954.

New York Times articles on proposed nuclear reactors in New York City. Includes Thirty Pickets Protest Plant for Queens Atomic Plant, November 12, 1963; Con Ed Withdraws Its Bid to Construct Atom Plant in City, January 7, 1964; Con Ed Planning Huge Atom Plant at Fort Slocum, July 25, 1968; Nuclear Plant Proposed Beneath Welfare Island, October 7, 1968; Con Ed Seeks to Build 2 Islands for Nuclear Power Plants Here, April 2, 1970.

Fuller J. We Almost Lost Detroit. New York: Ballantine Books, 1976.

Jablon S at al. Cancer in Populations Living Near Nuclear Facilities. National Cancer Institute. NIH Pub. No. 90-874, 1990.

U.S. Atomic Energy Commission. The Nation's Energy Future. Report delivered to President Richard Nixon, December 1, 1973.

Hatch MC et al. Cancer near the Three Mile Island nuclear plant: radiation emissions. American Journal of Epidemiology 1990;132(3):397-412.

U.S. Environmental Protection Agency, Office of Radiation Programs. Environmental Radiation Data. Montgomery AL. Quarterly reports.

E. Petridou et al. Infant leukemia after in utero exposure to radiation from Chernobyl. Nature 1996;382:352-3.

Michaelis J et al. Infant leukemia after the Chernobyl accident. Nature 1997;387:246.

Mangano JJ. Childhood leukemia in U.S. may have risen due to fallout from Chernobyl.

British Medical Journal 1997;304(7088):1200.

Scholz R. Ten Years After Chernobyl: The Rise of Strontium-90 in Baby Teeth. New York: International Physicians for the Prevention of Nuclear War, 1997.

Stamoulis KC et al. Strontium-90 concentration measurements in human bones and teeth in Greece. The Science of the Total Environment 1999;229:165-82.

Kulev Y et al. Strontium-90 concentrations in human teeth in South Ukraine, 5 years after the Chernobyl accident. The Science of the Total Environment 1994;155:215-9.

Chapter 8
Enstrom JE. Cancer mortality patterns around the San Onofre nuclear power plant, 1960-1978. American Journal of Public Health 1983;73(1):83-92.

Johnson CJ. Cancer and infant mortality around a nuclear power plant. American Journal of Public Health 1983;73(10):1216.

Pulley B. State to Study Ocean County Over Cancer. The New York Times, March 12, 1996.

New Jersey Department of Health and Senior Services. Case-Control Study of Childhood Cancers in Dover Township (Ocean County), New Jersey. Trenton NJ, 2001.

Breast cancer data in Suffolk County NY from National Cancer Institute. Published in Gould JM et al. The Enemy Within: The High Cost of Living Near Nuclear Reactors. New York: Four Walls Eight Windows, 1996.

Barry D and Revkin AC. At 50, Brookhaven Lab is Beset by Problems. The New York Times, March 22, 1997.

Groocock G. Radiation: Is Your Child in Danger? Suffolk Life Newspapers, Sufolk County NY, June 2, 1999.

Breast Cancer Mythology on Long Island. Editorial in the New York Times, August 31, 2002.

Kolata G. Epidemic That Wasn't. The New York Times, August 29, 2002.

Dreifus C. New Chief at Physics Lab Tries to Polish Faded Star. The New York Times, October 21, 2003.

Chapter 9
Personal correspondence, Ernest Sterrnglass, October 28, 2005.

O'Donnell RG et al. Variations in the concentration of plutonium, strontium-90 and total alpha-emitters in human teeth collected within the British Isles. The Science of the Total Environment 1997;201:235-43.

Personal correspondence, Hari Sharma, October 20, 2006, October 22, 2006.

Cimisi J. What Teeth May Tell Us. Dan's Papers, Southampton NY, June 11, 1999.

Gould JM et al. Strontium-90 in deciduous teeth as a factor in early childhood cancer. International Journal of Health Services 2000;30:515-39.

Margo Frances, email correspondence, January 19, 2007.

Klein M. Actor Pulling for Tooth Project. Westchester Journal-News, November 3, 2000.

Montgomery County (PA) Health Department. Investigation of Cancer Incidence in the Tri-County Greater Pottstown Area. Norristown PA, January 22, 1998.

Mangano JJ. Update on 1998 Report, Cancer Incidence in Greater Pottstown Area. September 5, 2002.

Mangano JJ et al. An unexpected rise in strontium-90 in US deciduous teeth in the 1990s. The Science of the Total Environment 2003;317:37-51.

Stoller G. Baby Teeth Offer Radioactive Clues. USA Today, January 2, 2004.

Chapter 10
Environmental Protection Agency, information on superfund sites by U.S. state. Available at www.epa.gov.

Tichler J et al. Radioactive Materials Released from Nuclear Power Plants. Upton NY: Brookhaven National Laboratory. NUREG/CR-2907. Prepared for U.S. Nuclear Regulatory Commission, annual reports, 1970-1993.

Emissions from nuclear reactors during 2001-04 available at www.reirs.com/emissions.

Cancer incidence data available at http://wonder.cdc.gov, national association of cancer registries.

Smothers R. Unable to Sell Nuclear Plant, Utility Seeks to Close It. The New York Times, July 9, 1998.

Sullivan J. Search for Cause of Cancer Cluster Yields Fear and Doubt. The New York Times, April 20, 1996.

Alec Baldwin comment made at Ocean County Community College, Toms River NJ. From Associated Press report, November 10, 1999.

Personal correspondence, Edith Gbur, October 27, 2006.

Personal correspondence, Barbara Bailine, November 2, 2006.

Corda J. State Extracts Funds for Tooth Fairy Project. The Southern Ocean (NJ) News, July 12, 2000.

Michael Harris, statement at Hackensack University Medical Center press conference, Hackensack NJ, November 12, 2003.

Timins JK. Radiation in pregnancy. Journal of the New Jersey State Medical Society 2001;98(6):29-33.

Letter from New Jersey Commission on Radiation Protection Chief Julie K. Timins to New Jersey Governor James McGreevey, December 17, 2003.

Ashford NA. New scientific evidence and public health imperatives. New England Journal of Medicine 1987;316(17):1084-5.

Letter from New Jersey Commission on Radiation Protection Chief Julie K. Timins to New Jersey Governor Jon Corzine, January 18, 2006.

Governor Opposed License. The New York Times, July 29, 2004.

Bowman D. Corzine a Skeptic on Plant, Tax. Gov Opposes 20-year Renewal of Oyster Creek's License. The Asbury Park (NJ) Press, August 4, 2006.

Chapter 11

Newman A. In Baby Teeth, a Test of Fallout. The New York Times, November 11, 2003.

Matthews C. Expanded Tooth Study Requested. The Westchester Journal News, Putnam and North Edition, February 22, 2001.

Lutzker L. Tooth Fairy Project Opposes A-Plant on Pseudo-Research. The Asbury Park (NJ) Press, February 1, 2004.

Ivry B. Tooth Study Ties Oyster Creek, Cancer In Kids. Hackensack (NJ) Record, January 4, 2005.

Louria DB. Health Risk One Reason to Close Oyster Creek. Asbury Park (NJ) Press, February 3, 2005.

Kanaracus C. Cutting Their Teeth: The Radiation and Public Health Project is Still Waiting for a State Grant. Westchester Weekly, July 6, 2001.

Klein M. Westchester Official Dismisses Cancer Study. The Westchester Journal News, August 22, 2003.

U.S. Nuclear Regulatory Commission, available at www.nrc.gov

Nuclear Energy Institute, available at www.nei.org.

Gentzel J. ACE: Study Shows 'Potential Link' to Radiation, Cancer. Pottstown (PA) Mercury, November 20, 2003.

Chapter 12
Pecher C et al. Radio-calcium and radio-strontium metabolism in pregnant mice. Proceedings of the Society for Experimental Biology and Medicine. 1941(46):91-4.

Haller O and Wigzell H. Suppression of natural killer cell activity with radioactive strontium: effector cells are marrow dependent. The Journal of Immunology 1977;118(4):1503-6.

Emmanuel FXS et al. Mice treated with strontium 90: an animal model deficient in NK cells. British Journal of Cancer 1981;44:160-5.

Committee on the Biological Effects of Ionizing Radiation. Health Risks from Exposure to Low Levels of Ionizing Radiation: BEIR VII. National Academy of Sciences, Washington DC, 2005.

National Cancer Institute. Estimated Exposures and Thyroid Doses Received by the American People from Iodine-131 in Fallout Following Nevada Atmospheric Nuclear Bomb Tests. Washington DC: U.S. Department of Health and Human Services, 1997.

Sharp L et al. Incidence of childhood brain and other non-haematopoietic neoplasms near nuclear sites in Scotland 1975-94. Occupational and Environmental Medicine 1999;56(5):308-14.

Busby C and Cato MD. Death rates from leukemia are higher than expected in areas around nuclear sites in Berkshire and Oxford-shire. British Medical Journal 1997;315(7103):309.

Black RJ et al. Leukemia and non-Hodgkin's lymphoma: incidence in children and young adults resident in the Dounreay area of Carthness, Scotland in 1968-91. Journal of Epidemiology and Comm8unity Health 1994;48(3):232-6.

Draper GJ et al. Cancer in Cumbria and in the vicinity of the Sellafield nuclear installation, 1963-90. British Medical Journal 1993;306(6870):89-94.

Goldsmith JR. Nuclear installations and childhood cancer in the UK: mortality and incidence for 0-9 year-old children 1971-1980. Science in the Total Environment 1992;127(1-2):13-35.

Kinlen LJ et al. Contacts between adults as evidence for an infective origin of childhood leukemia: an explanation for the excess near nuclear establishments in west Berkshire? British Journal of Cancer 1991;64(3):549-54.

Ewings PD et al. Incidence of leukemia in young people in the vicinity of Hinkley Point nuclear power station, 1959-86. British Medical Journal 1989;299(6694):289-93.

Cook-Mozaffari PJ et al. Geographical variation in mortality from leukemia and other cancers in England and Wales in relation to proximity to nuclear installations, 1969-78. British Journal of Cancer 1989;59(3):476-85.

Roman E et al. Childhood leukemia in the West Berkshire and Basingstoke and North Hampshire District Health Authorities in relation to nuclear establishments in the vicinity. British Medical Journal (Clinical Research Edition) 1987;294(6572):597-602.

Forman D et al. Cancer near nuclear installations. Nature 1987;329(6139):499-505.

McLaughlin JR et al. Childhood leukemia in the vicinity of Canadian nuclear facilities. Cancer Causes and Control 1993;4(1):51-8.

Viel JF et al. Incidence of leukemia in young people around the La Hague nuclear waste reprocessing plant; a sensitivity analysis. Statistical Medicine 1995;14(21-22):2459-72.

Hoffman W et al. A cluster of childhood leukemia near a nuclear reactor in northern Germany. Archives of Environmental Health 1997;52(4):275-80.

Goldsmith JR. Childhood leukemia mortality before 1970 among populations near two United States nuclear installations. Lancet 1989;1(8641):793.

Mangano JJ et al. Elevated childhood cancer incidence proximate to U.S. nuclear power plants. Archives of Environmental Medicine 2003;58(2):74-82.

Mangano JJ. A short latency between radiation exposure from nuclear plants and cancer in young children. International Journal of Health Services 2006;36(1):113-35.

Mangano JJ et al. Infant deaths and childhood cancer reductions after nuclear plant closings in the United States. Archives of Environmental Health 2002;57(1):23-32.

U.S. Surgeon General. Smoking and Health: Report of the Advisory Committee to the Surgeon General of the Public Health Service. Washington DC: U.S. Government Printing Office, 1964.